PRIMARY CA

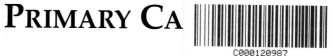

C000120987

AND

LABORATORY MEDICINE

A C B VENTURE PUBLICATIONS
with generous support from
Bayer (UK) Ltd
Boehringer Mannheim (UK) Ltd and MediSense Britain Ltd

Primary Care

and

Laboratory Medicine

EDITED BY:

JAMES HOOPER BSc, MB BS, MD, MRCPath.

Consultant Chemical Pathologist,
Royal Brompton Hospital,
London, UK.

GWYN McCREANOR BSc, MSc, PhD, MRCPath.

Principal Biochemist,
Royal Free Hospital,
London, UK.

WILLIAM MARSHALL MA, PhD, FRCP, FRCPath.

Senior Lecturer in Chemical Pathology,
King's College School of Medicine and Dentistry
London, UK.

PAUL MYERS MB BS, BSc, FRCGP, DRCOG.

General Practitioner,
Western Road Medical Centre,
Romford, UK.

FOREWORD BY:

ROGER HIGGS MBE, MA, FRCP, FRCGP

Professor of General Practice,
King's College School of Medicine and Dentistry,
London, UK.

A C B V E N T U R E P U B L I C A T I O N S

ACB VENTURE PUBLICATIONS

Chairman and Managing Editor - David Burnett.

British Library Cataloguing in Publication Data.

A catalogue record for the book is available from the British Library.

ISBN 0 902429 08 6 ACB Venture Publications

Design and Illustration – Michael Cartwright and Helen Morrison

Printed by Piggot Printers (Cambridge) Ltd.

Foreword

Change is a major part of clinical care in general practice. Our patients' needs and our own medical responses may alter as we get older together. Science and technology move, and the service changes in response to medical progress or political whim. Most clinicians have become familiar with the need to update themselves regularly about drugs, but fewer may realise that their use of the laboratory needs regular review. Laboratories themselves also need a routine way to check with practitioners if the service they are offering is what is required. This dialogue, and the adjustment of clinical and laboratory practice which go with it, is the focus of the book.

GPs share with laboratory specialists the burden of being expected somehow to know something about everything. Professionals achieve their own satisfaction in this impossible situation in different ways, but I cannot imagine a GP, who gives adequate time to his or her practice, who could not at the same time benefit from reading this book. Have it as a routine reference to hand, both to check on what is already being done and as a stimulus to better practice.

It is not easy to see exactly what the future will be for any part of healthcare, and certainly not for general practice, but some trends stand out when we look back. One of these has been the disappearance of the general physician and the increasing need for GPs not only to do the primary sorting but also the critical and detailed directing of those patients who do need specialised care. The mantle of the general physician has thus fallen on the doctor in the surgery; the GP and the laboratory specialist together need to make initial assessments, either in order to initiate the process of transfer to specific area of secondary care or to continue the investigation and monitoring of the patient's progress in general practice. This model, which pre-existed the new contract but has been underlined by it, requires the link between practice and laboratory to be of the very best.

There is a huge amount to learn here, and much that will fascinate. Its authors are to be congratulated on filling a much needed gap so well, and in providing a point of reference which is also a source of broad enlightenment.

Professor Roger Higgs

Preface

Laboratories provide vital services for primary care and such work will inevitably increase with the moves to increase the extent to which patients are treated in the primary care setting, an increase in day-case surgery and shorter in-patient stays. The relationship between laboratories and primary care should be a partnership with both the parties communicating efficiently in the interest of the patient.

This book is designed to help build on relationships already existing and stimulate others. It has been written to indicate how those in primary care may make the most effective use of the laboratory and to help those working in laboratories appreciate the nature of primary care work. Some general chapters describing the case-mix of primary care, the provision of service and interpretation of results are followed by discipline-specific chapters describing laboratory investigations and their interpretation. The book is meant to be used as a resource for rational laboratory investigation and the index is designed to reflect this with sections on clinical conditions and laboratory investigations.

In a working environment which seems to be increasingly crowded with commitments, one may wonder what motivates those wishing to write books. The production of a book which may be used both in primary care and in the laboratory should help all of us to provide a high-quality, cost-effective service for patients. The contributors and editors are grateful for the tolerance, encouragement and forbearance of colleagues (including secretaries), friends and families who helped bring this book to fruition.

May 1996
JH, GMc,WJM and PM

ACKNOWLEDGEMENTS

The editors are grateful to the following for their permission to reproduce or adapt material for certain figures used in this publication:

Pathology Departments, Havering Hospitals NHS Trust, Essex (Figure 2.3)

Blackwell Scientific Publication, Oxford. Fraser CG. Interpretation of clinical chemistry laboratory data. 1986 (Figure 3.10).

Dr Elizabeth Higgins, Senior Lecturer in Dermatology, King's College Hospital, London (Histopathology photographs used in Chapter 4).

CONTRIBUTORS

SALLY C. DAVIES MSc, MB, FRCP, MRCPath

Consultant Haematologist,
Central Middlesex Hospital,
London, UK.

JAMES HOOPER BSc, MB BS, MD, MRCPath.

Consultant Chemical Pathologist,
Royal Brompton Hospital,
London, UK.

STEPHEN HUMPHREYS BSc, MB, FRCPath

Consultant Pathologist,
King's College Hospital,
London, UK.

WILLIAM MARSHALL MA, PhD, FRCP, FRCPath.

Senior Lecturer in Chemical Pathology,
King's College School of Medicine and Dentistry
London, UK.

PAUL MYERS MB BS, BSc, FRCGP, DRCOG.

General Practitioner,
Western Road Medical Centre,
Romford, UK.

JOHN PHILPOTT-HOWARD MB, DCM, FRCPath

Senior Lecturer and Honorary Consultant Microbiologist,
King's College School of Medicine and Dentistry,
London, UK.

KATE RYAN MD, MRCP, MRCPath

Consultant Haematologist,
Central Middlesex Hospital,
London, UK.

ROMIL SAXENA MB, MRCPath

Lecturer in Histopathology,
King's College Hospital,
London, UK.

Contents

Chapter 1

Primary Care

Paul Myers

INTRODUCTION

There have been enormous changes in primary care since the introduction of the 'new contract' in 1990. In addition to alterations in the terms of service for General Practitioners (GPs) there has been a change in attitude to the provision of health care within the National Health Service (NHS). There is considerable evidence of the increasing integration between primary and secondary care. Examples of implementing this include changes in many areas of the provision of health care such as the use of joint clinical guidelines, improved communication between hospitals and GPs, and the introduction of collaborative audits.

These changes have been made in parallel with the introduction of an NHS broadly driven by market forces. Thus the introduction of 'purchasers' such as District Health Authorities and Fund Holding Practices, who contract clinical services from 'providers' such as Hospital Trusts and Community Units has brought with it many changes in the way service is provided. This has affected every area of clinical practice within the NHS, and has particular relevance in the interface between Laboratory Medicine Services and General Practice.

Until recently there was very little information available as to how many laboratory investigations were being requested by GPs, and little assessment as to the benefit in relation to cost, or to what extent the investigations influenced clinical management. It is well known that there appear to be wide variations in the number and type of laboratory tests that individual GPs request.

In some practices GPs have begun to perform some of these tests themselves, and the availability of new technology has widened the range of tests available in Primary Care. Since the introduction of fund holding, many practices have for the first time had the choice between NHS laboratories, those within the private sector, and near patient testing.

Thus the next few years are likely to see a more critical appraisal of the differential use of laboratory investigations between primary and secondary care. There have been calls for laboratories to become more responsive to the needs of General Practice, and this includes the provision of help in the presentation and interpretation of results.

The General Practitioner always has the responsibility to understand the relevance of a test result and, where appropriate, to investigate further or to refer, irrespective of where the test has been done. Therefore a GP's local laboratory can also be of assistance in these areas. It follows that GPs are likely to become increasingly involved in decision making in these areas of service provision. Increasing GP involvement is likely in the management of areas such as specimen collection, the delivery and format of laboratory results and to some extent quality control issues too. These issues may be specified by contract, and quality objectives are increasingly being included in contracts between providers and purchasers.

THE POSITION OF PRIMARY CARE WITHIN THE NATIONAL HEALTH SERVICE.

Every resident of the UK is entitled to healthcare provided by the National Health Service. The provision of NHS healthcare is organised into two principle sectors: primary care covers general medical , dental, ophthalmic and pharmaceutical services; secondary care covers hospital, ambulance, community, and specialised medical and nursing services. In addition mental health, care of the elderly and other community care is sometimes regarded as part of secondary care, and sometimes designated as part of tertiary care, as are specialised units often organised on a regional basis.

Responsibility for providing primary care lies with the 98 Family Health Service Authorities (FHSAs) in England and Wales and the 19 Health Boards in Scotland and Northern Ireland; however from April 1996 onwards the district health authorities and FHSAs will merge to form 'joint commissions' which will be responsible for both primary and secondary care.

GPs act as independent contractors with their local FHSAs and are usually the first point of contact for those requiring medical care. The UK is unique in that over 98% of the population is registered with a GP, from whom continuity of care may be directed. The great majority of GPs operate in group practices, and there is a progressive decrease in the percentage of single handed GPs, although these still make up a large proportion of inner city and urban practices. According to published Government expenditure plans the total NHS budget in the year to March 1995 was over £35 billion. Of this over £8.5 billion was allocated to the provision of primary care.

GENERAL PRACTICE PROFILE

THE WORKLOAD OF GENERAL PRACTICE

It is of interest to look at the 'Levels of Care' within the health system in the United Kingdom. Approximately 70% of all ill health in the UK is dealt with by self care, made up roughly as shown in Figure 1.1

Of the remaining medical problems which patients do not treat themselves, more than 90% are dealt with by GPs, and fewer than 10% by hospitals.

- 25% upper respiratory infections
- 20% rheumatological problems
- 20% psychological problems
- 10% gastrointestinal problems
- 5% skin problems
- 20% assorted problems

Figure 1.1   Self treated medical problems

There is a trend towards smaller list sizes in primary care. The average has been falling steadily, and there is a wide regional variation, with inner cities and urban areas having higher lists, and rural GPs having the lowest. The current UK average is about 1,900 patients per doctor.

In the UK, of the total of about 85,000 practising doctors, 30,000 are General Practitioners. These practice from about 9,000 surgeries, a quarter of which are purpose-built health centres. About 10% of GPs are dispensing GPs, practising in rural areas where pharmacies are scarce. These GPs provide a joint prescribing and dispensing role. Currently, about one quarter of all GPs are in the Fund Holding Scheme, and about a quarter of all practices are 'training practices' with a GP trainee in post.

The average doctor-patient contact rate is approximately 4.0 consultations per year. Again there is a wide regional variation, with urban areas, areas of deprivation, and those with a high elderly population tending to have higher rates.

The average surgery consultation time is estimated to be about 8 minutes, but GPs tend to show a very wide range in their consulting behaviour.

There is an average of 1 to 1.5 home visits per patient each year, although there has been a gradual reduction in the percentage of patients who are visited in their own homes. Approximately two thirds of any practice population tend to be seen over any one year period with 90% being seen over 5 years.

There is an increasing trend for GPs to practise within the structure of a Primary Health Care Team (PHCT). In this system GPs work closely with other Health Professionals, including attached staff such as District Nurses, Health Visitors and Midwives, as well as directly employed ancillary staff such as Nurse Practitioners, Practice Nurses, reception staff and administrators.

Since the introduction of contractual changes in 1990 the workload of GPs has increased considerably. There is much evidence that this is particularly related to administration, but with targets and an emphasis on health promotion the clinical side of General Practice has also increased significantly. For example, there has been an increase in practice-based health promotion programmes in the form of both well person clinics and opportunistic screening. In addition, there has been an increase in clinics dealing with the management of chronic disease in primary care. Other areas such as minor surgery, childhood immunisation, and child health surveillance have reflected the increasing transfer of clinical work from secondary to primary care.

A recent survey has shown that average GPs divide their work time as shown in Figure 1.2. The average surgery consultation in this survey was found to be 8.5 minutes.

Work area	Time (%)
Surgery consultations	44
Home visits including travelling	20
Patient case work	13
Administration	9
Attendance at special clinics (e.g., OPD)	3
Reading	4
Attending courses	3
Other	4

Figure 1.2   Division of GP's time

THE CLINICAL CONTENT OF GENERAL PRACTICE

Overall 65% of disorders seen in General Practice are minor and/or self-limiting. A further 15% of disease presentations are major or life-threatening and 20% of consultations relate to chronic disease and patients with permanent disability.

Over the last decade there has been a move in primary care from the basic treatment of acute illness, and chronic disease management to other activities relating to screening and health promotion.

Today a greater proportion of a GP's time is taken up with the monitoring of chronic diseases such as asthma, hypertension, chronic obstructive airways disease and ischaemic heart disease. Other clinical areas which previously were the domain of the GP are increasingly being delegated to ancillary staff, particularly practice nurses. These include procedures such as immunisations and wound care, as well as some chronic disease management.

It is usually accepted that 20% of the population are seen in a hospital outpatient department (OPD) in any one year. One of the principal roles of the GP is to act as a gate keeper to secondary care. An average GP makes 400 new referrals to hospital outpatient departments each year, but in fact only 5% of GP consultations lead to such referrals. In other words, the vast majority of medical problems that require medical attention are seen in primary care, and most are dealt with without the need for referral.

When considering the demand for laboratory investigations in primary care it may be useful to look at the prevalence of different diseases seen by General Practitioners. Figure 1.3 gives a range of conditions which may be seen in an 'average' practice of the equivalent of five full time GP principals looking after a medical list of 10,000 patients. However, there is no such thing as an 'average' practice, and when using the data for comparative purposes, corrections for the list size and special characteristics of the practice profile must be taken into consideration.

Note that in some cases the data relate to new patient episodes, and in others are consultations for the review of known disease. However the data are useful as a guide to the relative prevalence of different disorders. The data given were compiled from various sources including audits of a number of large group practices, including that of the author, as well as standard texts.

Births and Deaths

120 births:	116 in hospital and 4 at home		
100 deaths made up of:	4 infant deaths	32 coronaries	20 cancers
	16 strokes	4 accidents	24 others

Of these 25% of deaths occur at home, 65% in hospital and 10% elsewhere such as nursing home, public places, etc.

Minor Illness

2400	upper respiratory tract infections	1300	emotional disorders
800	gastrointestinal disorders	750	tonsillitis
300	otitis media	100	otitis externa
200	urinary tract infections	200	acute back pain
200	glandular fever		
60	sexually transmitted diseases (mainly gonorrhoea / non specific urethritis)		
10	infectious hepatitis		

Major Illness

400	acute bronchitis	80	pneumonias
40	coronary thrombosis	20	cerebro-vascular accidents
40	severe depression	20	new cancers diagnosed
25	renal colic	15	acute appendicitis
1	suicide		

Figure 1.3   Prevalence data for a practice of 10,000 patients

---

Chronic Illness

1000	chronic mental illness	1000	assorted joint problems
600	acute back problems	400	chronic rheumatisms
250	established asthma	200	chronic bronchitis
120	congestive cardiac failure	50 - 100	diabetics
80	iron deficiency anaemia	70	anaemias of other causes
60	rheumatoid arthritis	50	hypothyroidism
50	new coronary artery disease	40	epilepsy
30	new asthma	20	peptic ulcer disease
20	gout	12	pernicious anaemia
3 - 4	new hyperthyroidism	2	multiple sclerosis

Less than 1 new case of chronic renal failure per year.

Social Pathology

800	patients on welfare benefit	280	physically handicapped patients
160	unemployed patients	120	mentally handicapped patients
120	single parent families	100	deaf patients
40	blind patients	40	alcoholics
20	schizophrenics		

Newly Diagnosed Cancers

4	breast	2 - 3	colorectal
2 - 3	skin	2	lung
2	stomach	2	prostate
1	cervix	1	ovary every 6 years
1	leukaemia every 5 years	1	larynx every 6 years
1	uterus every 7 years		
1	primary brain tumour every 10 years		
1	lymphoma every 15 years		
1	thyroid cancer every 20 years		

Figure 1.3   Prevalence data for a practice of 10,000 patients

Congenital Disorders	
1 cardiac disorder every 5 years	1 pyloric stenosis every 7 years
1 spina bifida every 7 years	1 Down's syndrome every 10 years
1 cleft palate every 20 years	
1 congenital hip dislocation every 20 years	
1 phenylketonuria every 200 years	

Figure 1.3   **Prevalence data for a practice of 10,000 patients**

THE ROLE OF THE PRACTICE NURSE

The role of the practice nurse has been expanded and has changed significantly in the years since the introduction of the new contract for GPs. This has been partly driven by the new responsibilities and obligations that have been introduced, such as elderly person checks, health promotion targets, and immunisation targets. In particular there has been an enormous increase in data collection, and there has been a pressure on GPs to delegate many of the clinical and administrative tasks related to these clinical activities to their practice nurses. This has paralleled a trend of practice nurses seeking to increase their responsibilities and independence. In a number of more progressive practices the practice nurses are taking on a wider and more structured role including areas previously only considered the domain of the Medical Practitioner. Suitably trained practice nurses have developed this aspect into the role of the Nurse Practitioner, and these health professionals are not only taking on more work in chronic disease management and the screening of the practice population, but also are undertaking first visits in cases of acute illness.

Practice nurses have for many years been involved in the taking of clinical samples, and in most practices, venesection and the collection of MSUs and bacteriological swabs will be the responsibility of the practice nurses. Other traditional roles such as the provision of first aid and emergency treatment and advice as well as the application of dressings and the undertaking of minor procedures such as ear syringing and the removal of foreign bodies are well known. However, the extended nurse roles are beginning to include diagnostic and assessment procedures. These can only integrate satisfactorily with the role of the GP and other members of the Primary Health Care Team, as well as with the Hospital Service, through increasing multi-disciplinary collaboration, for example with regular team meetings and the more widespread use of regional clinical guidelines. In summary, it is likely that Nurse Practitioners will develop an extended role in clinical assessment and diagnosis and their greater involvement in the use of laboratory investigations is to be expected.

THE GP/HOSPITAL INTERFACE

About 1 in 9 of the population is admitted to hospital in any one year, and it has been estimated that up to 1 in 3 patients receive some kind of hospital care each year. Referral rates of patients from General Practice to hospital vary enormously between different practices and even between different doctors in the same practice. They can vary from 5 to over 100 patients per 1000 NHS patients per month. The reasons for this variation are multifactorial and include such diverse factors as the demography and case mix of the practice population, the provision of ancillary staff, access to direct hospital services, as well as the experience and ability of the GP, and the willingness to use laboratory services when available.

There has always been a wide range of management decisions in primary care, but the changes in the NHS are now resulting in pressures to change GP behaviour. For example, prior to the introduction of fund holding, and the various commissioning initiatives now evolving, a GP faced with a case of suspected renal colic could refer the patient to their local hospital for all investigations. Some GPs may have negotiated with the hospital for direct access to initial investigations including biochemistry, haematology, contrast radiology etc., although many GPs would have found it less time-consuming to make a direct urology referral. The major factors influencing the extent of GPs' involvement in investigating patients themselves would be their motivation, job satisfaction and abilities. Nowadays cost-effectiveness has been introduced as another pressure, and Fund Holding GPs in particular are finding that expansion of their role in investigating clinical problems directly often leads to increased patient convenience, cost savings and an increase in overall efficiency.

This has an important implication for the provision of and accessibility to hospital investigations. Access to a full range of laboratory investigations, as has now expanded through the Fund Holding scheme, means that GPs are no longer constrained by local policies which previously restricted the type and number of investigations. They may now arrange a full range of investigations wherever they wish, and although many will be dealt with under the block contract system, in theory, any investigation may be arranged by a Fund Holding GP.

The consequence of this open access is that, in theory, GPs will be able to avoid sending patients to OPD clinics purely for investigations, and time and expense could be saved by the GPs undertaking the organisation of these tests themselves.

THE REQUESTING & INTERPRETATION OF LABORATORY TESTS BY GPs

It is generally recognised that clinical information is often a more powerful predictor of clinical outcome than the results of batches of investigations, and this is probably more true in General Practice than any other speciality. However, the logical extension of assessing a patient by considering their signs and symptoms is by the support of appropriate investigations. The standard model in both primary and secondary care is to arrange investigations to support or refute clinical conjecture, or to distinguish between differential diagnoses. However, particularly in primary care, clinical assessment will often suggest the absence of organic disease, and then the demonstration of the absence of disease by investigation may be a powerful tool in reassuring the patient.

Many GPs will recall their years as house officers when they were expected to arrange mindlessly lists of tests so as to 'work up' a patient. Today, GPs are likely to look much more critically at how and why they investigate their patients. The extent to which patients are investigated by their GPs varies, reflecting the personalities and cultural backgrounds of both the GP and the patient, together with a multitude of other factors.

There are many pressures on GPs to increase their use of laboratory investigations, including an increasing saturation of the public with medical information by the media, often leading to misconceptions and inappropriate expectations of the provision of medical care within the NHS. There are other pressures on the GP too. For example, patients known to be at risk of inherited disease are increasingly being advised to enter screening schemes for such diseases. An increasing number of patients are being encouraged to demand screening procedures for occult disease, partly driven by the increase in consumerism, and the Government's various patients' charters. Most GPs have noticed an increasingly demanding group of patients - the 'worried well' - which consists of asymptomatic patients requesting investigations for as yet undiagnosed conditions.

Most GPs have their share of 'heartsink' patients; those chronic frequent attenders who generate multiple hospital referrals and investigations. There are a number of well recognised, albeit often unsatisfactory methods of terminating consultations with such patients, the classic one being the tendering of a prescription. However, other techniques employed by GPs may include the offer of a simple investigation such as a blood count, to conclude the consultation. Thus, sometimes GPs will order a test not so much to get information as to postpone a decision, i.e., to use time as a diagnostic or therapeutic tool, rather than use the test to define the problem. The use of these techniques is a part of normal General Practice, and it is helpful for their role in current practice to be recognised.

Other pressures on GPs to investigate patients include fear of litigation, although the increasing use of guidelines and protocols may introduce a more acceptable form of defensive medicine in which GPs will have a clear idea of what can be adopted as 'acceptable practice'. Increasing the collaborative work between primary and secondary care, and the evolution of shared clinical guidelines, and clinicians staffing pathology laboratories may have a key role in this area.

These pressures and the variation between practices have led to a wide qualitative and quantitative variation in GP behaviour with respect to choosing laboratory investigations. It may be anticipated that certain developments over the next few years will lead to a greater uniformity in the use of the Pathology Laboratory. In particular, this may result from the increasing drive for greater cost-effectiveness and the increase in structured education programmes for GPs. However, the greatest influence on the more judicious use of the laboratory may result from the increasing use of appropriate locally based Clinical Guidelines (or 'protocols'). This can result in the making of more appropriate and cost-effective clinical decisions, as well as preventing the duplication of work between primary and secondary care.

There are a number of questions that the GP, in common with any other clinician, should consider before undertaking a clinical investigation. First, one should carefully consider the clinical condition itself. Generally, the test should be specifically requested to confirm a clinical suspicion, with a view to altering the management of the patient to obtain a clinical benefit. A test should not be done simply to identify a group of patients with an abnormal result. A classical example of this inappropriate use of laboratory investigations arose at the peak of the popularity of Health Promotion Clinics introduced in the early 1990's. Here indiscriminate screening of practice populations led to reports of some practices succeeding in identifying cases of hypercholesterolaemia in patients aged over 90!

Second, the test should be arranged in the light of the natural history of the disorder. If this was self-limiting or trivial then the support of a presumptive diagnosis by investigation may be pointless. For example, most cases of acute diarrhoeal illnesses seen in General Practice are not investigated with stool cultures on presentation, as the majority of cases will have resolved by the time the results are available.

Third, the GP should have an approximate idea of the prevalence of the condition, together with the specificity and sensitivity of the test. Such knowledge will help the GP judge whether or not the test is likely to detect the disorder under suspicion.

Finally, and most importantly, the GP should have an idea as to how the result of the test would influence the management of the patient. Thus, a mid stream urine culture would be justified, even if blind treatment of a suspected urinary tract infection were to be offered immediately, since a change of antibiotic could be given based on the organism's sensitivities.

This concept is summarised in the much quoted advice:

'Before ordering a test decide what you will do if it is either positive or negative, and if both answers are the same, then don't do the test !'

With the expansion of laboratory investigations in primary care there are a number of areas which are becoming of increasing interest to GPs.

GPs will be looking to their local laboratories for comprehensive information on the following:

• *THE LABORATORY RESULT AND REFERENCE RANGE*
Obviously the reference range, which in many cases shows a wide variation between laboratories, is of crucial importance, and updated normal values should be easily

---

General Practitioners use their laboratory services in three main clinical areas:

- To diagnose and manage new disease presenting symptomatically, such as urinary tract infections, diabetes mellitus, rheumatoid arthritis, etc. Here the GP will anticipate that a higher proportion of the results will be positive, or in the abnormal range, than in the 'screening' group.

- To monitor chronic established disease: such as the review of patients with treated diabetes, hypothyroidism or hyperthyroidism, and chronic renal failure, as well as the monitoring of patients' plasma drug concentrations when treated with potentially toxic agents.

- To screen for subclinical disease, such as the cervical cytology scheme, and screening for iron deficiency anaemia in antenatal patients. Here the GP will anticipate that most of the results will be negative, or in the normal range.

Figure 1.4   The use of laboratory services by General Practitioners

accessible. For example, the values may need to be corrected for weight or body build. For more information concerning the reference range see Chapter 3.

• *FACTORS INFLUENCING THE RESULT.*
There are numerous factors which may alter the result of a laboratory test, and the average GP may not be familiar with the less well-known ones. The presence of physiological factors, concomitant disease or drug treatment may often be relevant. These can be divided into pre-analytical, analytical and post-analytical factors and are discussed in detail in Chapter 3. It is the responsibility of the laboratory to ensure that the GP is aware of such factors where applicable. Two-way communication is of crucial importance here; the laboratories will need to be given appropriate clinical details, as they could not be expected to know these otherwise, and GPs should be notified about interactions where relevant so that the results may be interpreted correctly.

• *EXPLANATION FOR ABNORMAL RESULTS*
Although the reason that a laboratory result is abnormal may be obvious, GPs are looking increasingly to their laboratories to provide additional information to help in the differentiation between health and disease. Laboratories can help the clinician by suggesting likely causes of abnormal profiles. For example, it is quite common for the report of an abnormal blood film showing atypical lymphocytes helpfully to refer to the possibility of glandular fever, and for the laboratory to initiate further tests, if possible with the original blood sample provided. Similar additional information may be appropriate in cases of abnormal lipid profiles, or liver function test results outside the normal range, etc.

• *INDICATIONS FOR OTHER INVESTIGATIONS*

Abnormal test results may suggest a further line of inquiry, and it can be time-saving to the GP if such information is made available for individual patients. For example, a haematological report of a megaloblastic blood film with a shift to the right might refer to the need for a follow up B_{12} and folate, to exclude pernicious anaemia.

• *TEST REQUESTS AND RESULTS*

The manner in which investigations are requested and the results fed back to the GP is subject to rapid change and innovation. The wider use of uniform request forms helps GPs to save time and allows more efficient use of resources. The use of the postal service or a local hospital courier service to send back results is now becoming outdated, and many laboratories will fax results back the same day as receiving the samples. This is only one step away from the recently introduced 'links' projects which allow laboratories to be linked electronically to GPs' surgeries via modems. The results may then be down-loaded electronically to a practice based computer system. The results would then find their way directly to the individual patient's record, so saving considerable time (p24).

WHAT LEVELS OF INVESTIGATIONS ORIGINATE IN PRIMARY CARE ?

Most laboratories will report a wide range of activity levels when different practices are compared with one another. There are many factors operating here, and there is no 'correct' level of activity with respect to any given GP or practice. For example, developed practices which have active health promotion programmes may tend to ask for a greater number and wider range of investigations. Group Practices may have fairly strict guidelines to control and monitor their investigations, and depending on their content this may either increase or decrease activity.

Probably the most important determinant in laboratory request variation is the population profile of the patients. Factors such as the age and sex distribution, social class and education of the patients may be crucial. For example, in an affluent area many patients may be investigated within the private sector, and so the request rate of tests within the NHS may appear relatively low. Many other factors also need to be considered; practices with a research interest may have screening programmes which will entail increased activity.

The increasing number of Fund Holding practices may see a change in the range and use of laboratory investigations in primary care. Thus in the future, if fiscal considerations are increasingly brought in to the equation, practices will be expected to become more discriminating in their choice of tests. A drive to keep within budget may increase the use of near patient testing for example, where certain tests are cheaper to arrange on the premises rather than at the local hospital.

Currently most Fund Holding practices cover the costs of pathology services by block contracts based on historical activity data. Provided the practices stay within a specified activity range they will remain within budget. This lessens the incentive for more innovation and selectivity in contract setting for pathology services. However in the medium term, downward pressure on a practice's fund may see a drive to greater cost-effectiveness in GP's choice of laboratory services.

Thus there are complex factors working in the requesting of laboratory investigations within the NHS. There can be no definitive investigation request rate for any one practice, any more than there can be an optimum number of hospital referrals or prescriptions issued by a GP.

Notwithstanding the wide range of investigation requirements between individual GPs and between different practices, and the factors that influence them, it may be useful to show the request rates for a typical suburban practice for a range of pathological services.

Data is given in Figures 1.5 - 1.10 which shows the annual request rates for a variety of laboratory investigations, given for an 'average' practice with a list size of 10,000 patients. Such data can be used for broad comparative purposes, but one should always consider the difficulties in comparing data from different General Practices which have already been mentioned.

Haematology	Number of Investigations
Full blood count	1100
ESR / viscometry	450
Blood group	150
Rubella TPHA titre	100
Paul Bunnell test	30
B_{12} and folate	25
Iron and ferritin	10
Miscellaneous haematology	130

Figure 1.5   Summary of Haematology investigations per annum for a practice of 10,000 patients

Biochemistry	Number of Investigations
Urea & electrolytes	620
Liver function tests	360
Cholesterol / lipids	350
Blood sugar	270
Uric acid	130
Glycated haemoglobin	120
Gamma glutamyl transferase	25
Amylase	20
Creatine kinase	20
Acid phosphatase / PSA	20
Miscellaneous biochemistry	30

Figure 1.6   Summary of Biochemistry investigations per annum for a practice of 10,000 patients

Therapeutic Drugs	Number of Investigations
Lithium	35
Digoxin	10
Phenobarbitone	10
Phenytoin	10
Carbamazepine	10
Theophylline	10
Miscellaneous drug levels	5

Figure 1.7 Summary of Therapeutic Drug investigations per annum for a practice of 10,000 patients

Endocrinology	Number of Investigations
Thyroid function	350
LH / FSH	110
Oestrogens	30
Testosterone	30
Prolactin	25
Sex hormone binding globulin	10
Miscellaneous endocrinology	90

Figure 1.8 Summary of Endocrinology investigations per annum for a practice of 10,000 patients

Immunology	Number of Investigations
C-reactive protein	65
Rheumatoid factor	60
Auto-antibodies	60
Antinuclear factor	40
Immunoglobulins	35
Miscellaneous immunology	15

Figure 1.9 Summary of Immunology investigations per annum for a practice of 10,000 patients

Microbiology / Histopathology	Number of Investigations
Mid-stream urine culture	320
High vaginal swab	65
Stool culture	40
Ear / nasal / throat swab	30
Wound swab	25
Miscellaneous bacteriology / virology	25
Histology	60

Figure 1.10   **Summary of Microbiology / Histopathology investigations per annum for a practice of 10,000 patients**

FURTHER READING

Fry J, Brooks D, McColl I. NHS Data Book. Lancaster: MTP Publications, 1994.

Fry J. Common Diseases. 5th Edition, Newbury: Kluwer Academic Publications, 1993.

Hodgkin K. Towards Earlier Diagnosis, Edinburgh: Churchill Livingstone 1993.

Stillwell B, Bowling A. The Changing Role of the Practice Nurse in the U.K. The Nurse in Family Practice. London: Scutari Press, 1988.

Hopkins A. Appropriate Investigation and Treatment in Clinical Practice. London: Royal College of Physicians 1989.

Chapter 2

Provision of Service

James Hooper

INTRODUCTION

The past few years have seen an enormous change in the way in which the delivery of health care is managed. With the emphasis on changing the pervading culture within the NHS to be more market-driven, the purchaser/provider split has placed great purchasing power on GPs, particularly fundholders. With purchasing power has come more direct access in determining the details of the costs of laboratory service provision and influence on what kind of service is offered and how it is delivered. The provision of service can be formalised by service specifications, which are becoming more detailed and specific as experience grows. This will almost certainly plateau soon, to give both purchasers and providers time to develop lasting relationships and possibly longer and more stable contracts.

A word of caution needs to be sounded, however, in response to some activities associated with market-driven service provision. Many demands upon laboratory service provision have and are being made on aspects of service which have no direct clinical relevance, especially in terms of speed and selection of tests. The change (in relation to pathology laboratories) from being passive players in the theatre of health care to active purchasers in the market-place can place GPs in positions so powerful that some aspects of service provision are being requested that have very little relevance to patient care e.g., the demand to decrease turnaround times for tests which do not alter the immediate management of patients and which may lead to increased test costs because of the increased frequency of analytical runs. Although there may be advantages in terms of making the providers (the laboratories) more responsive, attention must be given to the imperatives of clinical care.

Purchasers must be aware that pathology is a clinical speciality and that Consultant Pathologists have a vital role in helping to choose the correct tests for investigation, in suggesting other tests if they are more relevant and in interpreting the results of the tests in conjunction with general practitioners. In such a way, inappropriate tests may be avoided and more suitable ones suggested. Such help has an impact on cost-effectiveness, which is being increasingly scrutinised. It would be disastrous to good links that many hospital laboratories have made with local GPs if these were to be squandered on the basis of comments such as, "Well, I've ordered the test; if you don't do it for me, I'll go somewhere that can do it for me". It is therefore vital that such aspects of service, such as consultation, are specified in agreements if we are to avoid financial imperatives taking complete precedence over clinical ones.

It may be that users of the service have a stark choice: either to contract with a factory-type laboratory (results only), which will perform all requested tests and not even have the option of professional guidance and interpretation, or to contract with a consultant-led service, which provides 24-hour advice, but which may refuse requests which are inappropriate and suggest other, more relevant tests, together with helpful, interpretive advice. See Figure 2.6 for an example of a consultation between a GP and a Consultant Chemical Pathologist.

A more positive view, which is important in the provision of a high-quality service is the idea that the provision of service is in the form of a partnership between the GP-user and the laboratory-provider. For this to happen effectively depends upon good communication, so that trust and confidence can develop. Various aspects of the service, together with ways in which good communication can be effected, is given below in the section on Service Provision.

GP-SPECIFIC REQUIREMENTS

Pathology tests may be requested for a wide variety of reasons, ranging from diagnosis to safety documentation e.g., in connection with drug trials. The pattern of requesting is different for each pathology specialty, with histology tests particularly being targeted at diagnosis. In addition, the pattern of requesting is likely to be quite different for GPs than for hospital-based users. Pathology tests may be used as illustrated in Figure 2.1.

The use of pathology tests in general practice:

- to help establish diagnosis

- to help confirm or refute clinical diagnosis

- to distinguish between differential diagnoses

- to exclude disease

- to manage treatment

- to monitor the effectiveness of treatment

- to monitor the concentration of therapeutic agents

- to facilitate the early detection of disease

- to screen for disease

- to provide safety documentation.

Figure 2.1   Use of pathology tests

General practitioners use a fairly limited proportion of laboratories' repertoires and these tests are required mainly for monitoring disease and treatment or excluding disease and only occasionally for diagnosis. For example, although a mid stream urine sample may be required to confirm a diagnosis of urinary tract infection and skin biopsy required for some dermatological conditions, the bulk of tests requested are for monitoring treatment e.g., plasma potassium concentration in patients on diuretic therapy and blood glucose concentration in diabetes or a full blood count and erythrocyte sedimentation rate to exclude disease in patients with vague symptomatology (see Chapter 1).

In general, the turnaround time for such tests is not critical, although arrangements can be made for urgent requests. However, it is vital that GPs have confidence in the system which should perform consistently and to a high standard. It is vital that a GP can be sure that a result for plasma glucose, say, is reported back to the surgery before he next sees a diabetic patient whose insulin therapy may be difficult to control. Thus, the emphasis again is on good relationships, liaison and building a partnership which can be relied upon.

SERVICE PROVISION

The provision of laboratory services covers the whole process of the GP's choice of test in the appropriate circumstance, to carrying out the test in the laboratory and finally to the GP receiving a report of the test with interpretation where relevant. The separate, but linked, activities that comprise the service are examined below. The provision of a high-quality service is dependent on a number of factors, the most important of which is the relationship or partnership established between the GP and the laboratory.

A number of changes are taking place within laboratories, which may affect, and should help, the provision of an integrated pathology service. Within the UK, pathology services are traditionally divided into separate disciplines, each of which is responsible for its own particular branch of the service. Such a discipline-specific service is strengthened by the fact that staff (including medical staff) undergo discipline-specific training, although initial training is usually multi-specialty based. Two factors, however, are presently driving change. First, with increasing automation, certain aspects of the service (including some of each of biochemistry, haematology, immunology and microbiology) can be delivered from a single laboratory. Second, pressures on laboratories to be more cost-effective influence the way in which they operate and in particular, stimulate an integration of common activities e.g., specimen reception and reporting. These factors will increasingly influence the way in which pathology services are delivered.

LABORATORY INFORMATION

For a GP to make a suitable choice of tests, it is vital that he or she has easy access to up-to-date laboratory information. Ideally, this should be in the form of a handbook, which should include the information given in Figure 2.2.

- telephone numbers for laboratory (information and results; consultant advice)

- list of tests with reference ranges, specimen requirements and turnaround times

- safety information and how to collect specimens

- cost of tests (optional).

Figure 2.2   Contents of Laboratory Handbook

The most important aspect of such a handbook is that it should be user-friendly and this can be attained if laboratories listen to what GPs require for a service and modify existing information accordingly. Inevitably, time and energy are required to ensure this and once again, liaison is crucial. One aspect of the coming together of some laboratory functions, as mentioned above, is the fact that some laboratories are now providing a single telephone number for all result enquiries. This eases GPs' access to the laboratory. If at all possible, such numbers should be direct-dial lines.

REQUEST FORMS

Just as the laboratory's traditional organisation was based on separate departments, with separate enquiry points, most laboratories still have separate request forms for the various disciplines. This may help their internal organisation but is not user-friendly for GPs, who increasingly require that test-requesting is kept as simple as possible. It is not important for GPs to know which discipline, for example performs immunological tests - for these may be done, due to local circumstances, in biochemistry, microbiology, haematology or even immunology itself. What is vital is that the laboratory service is apparently seamless and acts in a co-ordinated manner.

It is also important to note that it may not be GPs who actually fill out request forms and thus ease of use is vital. Some hospital laboratories have designed a single pathology request form, which may be tailored to the needs of a particular practice user. Figure 2.3 is an example of a combined pathology request form.

HAVERING HOSPITALS	COMBINED PATHOLOGY REQUEST FORM	Please use a ball point pen

NHS No.	Drs. Hartley Myers Bass Leigh-Collyer Bond Haskell Western Road Medical Centre Romford, RM1 3LS Tel: 01708 746495 Fax: 01708 737936	Drop No. **102**
Surname		
Forenames		
Address	Relevant clinical details	
Postcode		
Sex D.o.B		High risk YES/NO

Type of Specimen: Blood   MSU   CSU   Faeces   Other   Private/NHS

BIOCHEMISTRY	HAEMATOLOGY	IMMUNOLOGY	MICROBIOLOGY
U&E	Full blood count	Rheumatoid factor	MC & S
Liver profile	Plasma Viscosity/ESR	Thyroid antibodies	AFB Culture
Bone profile	Paul Bunnell	Immunoglobulins	Parasitology
Glucose	Other	Antinuclear antibodies	Chlamydia
Total T4		Other	Mycology
Urine pregnancy test			Other
Cholesterol			
Other	For Laboratory use only		

Figure 2.3   Combined pathology request form

COLLECTION AND TRANSPORT OF SPECIMENS

Successful laboratory diagnosis depends greatly upon the selection, timing and method of collection of specimens. Medical staff are therefore encouraged to discuss with the laboratory any problem regarding the choice of investigation, the nature and the method of collection of specimens, and the interpretation of results.

PHLEBOTOMY

Samples may be taken by the GP, the practice nurse, health visitor or by a dedicated phlebotomist. Information and training are important, especially if it is not the GP taking the samples, since repetition of sampling due to an inappropriate or insufficient specimen is annoying, costly and causes delay to the clinical process. Some laboratories are able to provide phlebotomy services for local GPs, as part of a service agreement (contract) and as more GPs are becoming fundholders, many are now requesting this as part of an integrated pathology service. However, although this may be possibly in urban areas, geographical limitations may rule it out in rural practices.

COLLECTION AND HANDLING OF SPECIMENS

Venous blood, ideally taken by venepuncture, is preferred for most biochemical and haematological investigations. Blood taken by skin puncture or capillary methods is sometimes useful for paediatric samples or in cases of poor venous access, but may produce less reliable results, which are technique dependent.

TRANSPORT

Transport arrangements must be reliable if they are to be of use. Just as geographical position affects the provision of phlebotomy, so too may it dictate the transport of specimens (and reports). Many urban practices will receive regular and timed visits by a hospital courier service, collecting specimens and delivering reports and other materials. Evidently, other arrangements are also effective, as long as they are reliable e.g., a taxi service or delivery of specimens by practice staff. The key to a good transport service is excellent communication and organisation. Hospital transport drivers need to know exactly where to pick up specimens and to deliver goods and reports. Samples must be ready on time, since very often complex rounds are made and delays in one practice have knock-on effects on others. Although some transport arrangements have the facility for call-out for urgent specimens, such a provision may be costly. As with many aspects of pathology service provision, it is worth taking some time to determine a practice's exact needs when drawing up contracts.

LEAKAGES AND ACCIDENTS

If a specimen is seen to be leaking within its sealed compartment, but without contamination of the outside of the bag, the bag should be carefully placed within a second sealable plastic bag and sent to the laboratory for disposal. If other specimens and bags have become contaminated, they should be placed in a large plastic bag by a senior member of the clinic or surgery, using disposable plastic gloves. The large plastic bag should be tied or sealed and labelled "Contaminated - Danger of Infection", and sent to the laboratory for sorting and disposal. The laboratory should be notified by telephone. If a specimen is broken whilst in transit; no attempt should be made to salvage it or clear away glass, but the specimen must be taken to the receiving laboratory, which should be informed of the breakage.

Vacuum container needle holders

Medical and paramedical staff must discard the vacuum container plastic needle holders if they become contaminated with blood, in order to avoid the risk of cross-infection between patients.

Needle injuries

Discard all used needles and sharps safely, into a sharps bin, and never into plastic waste bags. Apart from the risk of exposing yourself and others to HIV and hepatitis viruses, an identified offender could face disciplinary action by the Health & Safety Executive. If a needlestick accident occurs or similar exposure to one of the inoculation-risk viruses, telephone a Medical Microbiologist or attend the Accident & Emergency Department. Even if the person involved has had hepatitis B vaccination, a booster dose of vaccine or immunoglobulin may be required. With regard to needle injuries involving a patient known or strongly suspected to have HIV, prophylactic antiviral drugs may be indicated and medical attention should be sought straight away.

REPORTS

Traditionally, laboratories have reported results using paper forms but other means of report delivery are being increasingly used e.g., facsimile and electronic links. The paper copy of the result is still the standard against which all other report formats must be compared and is at present the essential one for medicolegal purposes. The legality of electronic messaging alone as being the record of the result is presently being examined.

REPORT FORMS

For these to be useful, they have to be readable, timely and any comments must be relevant. Great care must be taken by the laboratory in the design of report forms, with the vital patient identifiers, requesting doctor and practice clearly shown. Where numerical results are given, these must be accompanied by reference ranges (age/sex related if possible) and abnormal results should be indicated by, for example, an asterisk or use of a different colour. Some laboratories are able to provide not only an emphasis of an abnormal numerical result but also automatic notification of a significant change from a previous one on the same patient. This notification of change is called a 'delta check' and the limits for it may be set by the laboratory e.g., if the plasma sodium concentration changes from a previous result in the same patient by more than, say, 8 mmol/L. Where text is included, this should be succinct, easy to understand and unambiguous. If, for example, the report is of a histological specimen, great care must be taken to identify the report as provisional if further tests are being carried out.

TELEPHONED RESULTS

In some circumstances, it is vital that the telephone is used to convey urgent, unexpected or very abnormal results e.g., high plasma glucose. Good communication is required for this and laboratories have to have in place effective ways of identifying such abnormal results and to know to whom results should be telephoned. For the GP, it is vital that the laboratory is aware of the telephone numbers to use in such circumstances, that receptionists are well-trained in receiving results and that they are immediately communicated to the relevant doctor. The possibility of transcription errors is a real concern and it is vital for both parties concerned to ensure that ambiguous numbers, e.g., 50 or 15, are clearly conveyed by words five zero or one five. The telephoned result must be repeated to the caller by the recipient, since this helps to avoid transcription errors. The final report coming from the laboratory must indicate that the results have been telephoned. Figure 2.4 is an example of a laboratory report.

FACSIMILE

Many laboratories now report results to outside users by facsimile and this trend is increasing. There are two areas of concern over such transmission:

Quality

A problem of confusion exists, particularly with some numerical results over certain digits e.g., '8' and '0' can look very similar on some facsimile print-outs. Care must be taken both with font and size chosen for the paper report that has to be transmitted. GPs must be aware of the possibility of digit confusion. Additionally, facsimile text fades over

ROYAL FREE HOSPITAL NHS TRUST

PATIENT	GENERAL PRACTICE	
SMITH ALICE	Dr A. Golden	Printed 05/02/96
11203654	225 Hampstead Hill	Time 1640
DOB 11 November 1930	Hampstead	Received 05/02/96
Age 65 years	London NW3	Page 1
Female		

Test	Result	Ref range	Units
Chemistry			
Sodium	142	(135 - 145)	mmol/L
Potassium	4.6	(3.6 - 5.0	mmol/L
Creatinine	75	(60 - 120)	μmol/L
Urea	4.5	(2.5 - 6.7)	mmol/L
TSH	**20.2 *c**	(0.3 - 5.0)	mU/L
fT$_4$	**<5.0 *c**	(10 - 26)	pmol/L
Haematology			
HB	**11.5 ***	(12.0 - 16.0)	g/dL
HCT	**34.1 ***	(36.0 - 46.0)	%
WBC	7.1	(4.5 - 11.0)	x10^9
RBC	**3.88 ***	(4.50 - 5.90)	x10^{12}
MCV	**110 ***	(81.0 - 99.0)	fL
MCH	29.6	(27.0 - 32.0)	pg
MCHC	33.7	(31.0 - 36.0)	%
Platelets	295	(150 - 400)	x10^9
Lymphocytes	1.7	(1.3 - 3.0)	x10^9
Neutrophils	4.4	(2.2 - 7.0)	x10^9
Eosinophils	0.2	(0.0 - 0.4)	x10^9
Monocytes	0.4	(0.2 - 0.8)	x10^9
Basophils	0.1	(0.0 - 0.1)	x10^9

Comment: The elevated TSH and suppressed fT4 indicate biochemical hypothyroidism. No indication of treatment was given on the request card and if the patient is known to be hypothyroid and is already on thyroid hormone replacement therapy then replacement is inadequate.

Dr P. Lasma, Principal Biochemist. 05/02/96.

Symbols used: * = outside reference range   c = comment.

Figure 2.4   Example of laboratory report

time on heat-sensitive paper and is not suitable as a filed report. Although a photocopy of the facsimile result may make a more permanent record, this process requires organisation and time. Plain facsimile paper gives a permanent record.

Confidentiality
Just as paper records are confidential, so too are transmitted facsimile results. Often, facsimile machines are placed in relatively public areas in practices and laboratories, and care must be taken to ensure confidentiality, by placing the facsimile machine in an appropriate place.

COMPUTER LINKS
There are currently a number of schemes employing electronic data interchange (EDI) to allow direct communication between laboratory computers and those in GP practices. The main benefits of electronically transmitting laboratory data are the availability of timely reports and the avoidance of re-keying information into the GP's computer system with the associated reduction in transcription errors. In addition, the electronic merging of reports into patient records based on demographics supplied in the original requests, reduces the possibility of reports being matched with the wrong patients.

The laboratory results are translated into a standard format in preparation for electronic transmission and sent via a modem on existing telephone lines to a message handling system which administers the mailboxes used to store and forward the information to the GP's surgery. The surgery also requires a modem attached to its computer system to allow communication over the telephone lines and allow receipt of the laboratory data. Confidentiality is ensured by the use of identification codes and passwords.

Clearly, the real advantages of EDI will only be realised when information can be fully integrated into the patient record. Few existing GP systems currently support this activity and even some systems currently under development are not being designed to fulfil this function. To overcome the lack of functionality in the existing systems, some software suppliers have developed stand-alone solutions that require a personal computer attached to a modem in the surgery and store the results in a proprietary database independently of the practice's computing system. Although limited in its usefulness, some GPs find this intermediate solution has the advantage of allowing priority review of laboratory results pending arrival of the paper report. See Figure 2.5 for an example of an electronic GP link.

URGENT ARRANGEMENTS
Although not frequently required, laboratories must be able to provide analysis of urgent specimens, particularly for biochemistry and haematology. Again, good communication is the key to an efficient service and the GP must have easy access to a named member of senior staff or a deputy who should always be available to liaise. Urgent transport of specimens may be made either by the laboratory or the GP, depending on the circumstances and existing transport arrangements. A contact number for the GP must be given to the laboratory, especially if the analysis will take place outside normal surgery hours.

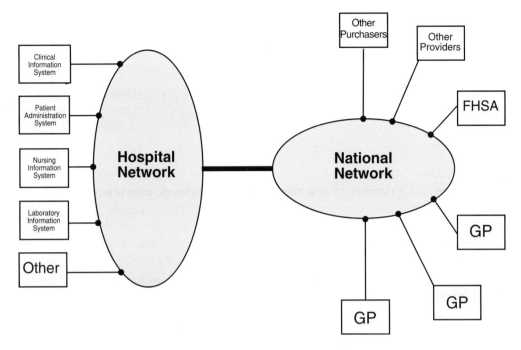

Figure 2.5   **Electronic GP links**

CONSULTANT ADVICE

All NHS laboratories should have departmental heads of Consultant status, who are available for advice and help. Advice may be sought on the choice of appropriate tests for investigating particular diseases or helping to narrow a differential diagnosis. Additionally, help may be required in the interpretation of more unusual test results or of unexpected or abnormal results. Such help should also be available out-of-hours and details of contact arrangements should be available in the laboratory handbook.

Consultant-led help may not be available in private laboratories or factory-type laboratories and this has to be considered when contracts are being drawn up, since test costs and hence contract prices will reflect the inclusion or otherwise of consultant advice.

Consultation Between a GP and a Consultant Chemical Pathologist.

GP

Hello, I wonder if you can help with a problem. Mr X, a 52-year old West Indian man has been treated by me for hyperlipidaemia for 2 years with simvastatin. I have heard that this type of drug can cause muscle problems, so I sent in a sample for CK analysis. It came back at 406 IU/L.

CONSULTANT

Yes, that's rather high - over twice the upper end of our reference range. I can see your concern. Is the patient well at present? In particular, does he have any muscle aches or chest pain?

GP

No, he appears quite well.

CONSULTANT

I am a little concerned since the statins can cause myositis. It is possible, however, that his high creatine kinase (CK) activity may not be drug-related.

GP

You don't think he's had an infarct, do you?

CONSULTANT

No, although it's an outside possibility and you ought to check with an ECG if you are concerned. The most likely reason is because of his ethnic background. West Indians, and the black population generally, often have higher CK activities than Caucasians. The reasons for this are not known and it is quite well recognised in the USA but less so here. I recommend that you stop his statin for 6 weeks and then repeat his CK measurement.

8 WEEKS LATER

GP

Thank you for your help with Mr X. His CK off simvastatin was 430 - it seems that the statin was not contributing. Is it safe to continue treatment with statin in this patient?

CONSULTANT

Yes, I think it is, although now having a benchmark CK for him, you might wish to measure his CK activity occasionally.

LEARNING POINTS

1.   If you are concerned about the interpretation of tests, ask your local hospital for advice - all laboratories should have access to consultant help.

2.   Measure CK activity before putting patients on statins.

Figure 2.6   **Consultation between a GP and a Consultant Chemical Pathologist**

QUALITY ASSURANCE

Quality assurance is about doing the job well and doing it only once - that is without having to repeat it. Many users of pathology services will know of the great amount of time (and money) that is spent by laboratories in assuring the quality of the analytical service, particularly for analyses that have numerical values. Additionally, much effort is expended in ensuring diagnostic accuracy by the circulation of slides for microscopic examination. As analytical instruments continually improve, the error tolerances for analyses become smaller and smaller and even greater effort is required to ensure that analyses are 'in control'. Users should be reassured by this effort and by the fact that laboratories invariably subscribe to independent quality assessment schemes.

Laboratories carry out two types of analytical quality assurance. First, internal quality control procedures involve the inclusion within analytical batches of patient samples, of material (internal quality control material) of known value or composition. Patient results are only accepted if the internal quality control material provides a value within a given narrow range. Second, external quality assessment schemes involve the analysis by the laboratories of material sent from coordinating national centres. Such samples are treated as if they were patient samples i.e., their value is not known. The results are sent back to the coordinating centre, which then provides information on the laboratory's performance in comparison with others, and provides a good measure of accuracy.

However, quality assurance is not just about quality control and quality assessment — it is about the whole process of providing an effective and efficient service. Total assurance of quality starts with the requesting doctor asking himself or herself the correct question e.g., is a laboratory test likely to be of help in this situation and if so, which tests should be used? The other elements of the service already described above then come into play, with the final elements being that of the delivery of the correct result on the correct patient back to the correct doctor at the correct time (and, if possible, supporting or refuting a clinical diagnosis). Although it is difficult to ensure that the whole system is working effectively, moves have been made to ensure that as many elements as possible in the total service are under scrutiny and are being controlled. The consideration of all the processes that comprise the service can be described by Total Quality Management — a means of control over quality which has been used in industry. Important elements of this process include attention to quality laboratory practices and quality improvement, as well as the more conventional quality control procedures.

Within the UK, a national laboratory accreditation scheme (Clinical Pathology Accreditation) has been established since 1992 and most laboratories are working towards becoming, or have become, accredited. The scheme has the support of the Department of Health, the Royal College of Pathologists and other professional organisations. Inspections are carried out by independent inspectors, who measure the laboratory's compliance against 44 nationally agreed standards covering the management of the laboratory and provision of a high-quality service. Only three of the standards are discipline-specific e.g., the provision of postmortem facilities, the rest being common to all disciplines. Inspectors also interview users of the service (hospital doctors and GPs), together with senior management of the hospital. Successful inspection allows the laboratories to be accredited and the process acts as an assurance of the quality of the total service.

As involvement within the scheme grows, purchasers are likely to require such a process within the contract specification. Although other forms of quality certification exist e.g., British Standard 5750 (ISO 9000), these do not necessarily measure laboratories' compliance with national standards.

In addition to the 44 standards covered in the accreditation process, many laboratories have become involved with the setting of local standards covering all aspects of laboratory service provision. These may be common to all laboratories e.g., the following up of queries within a given specified time, or be specific e.g., the reporting of 95% of urgent specimens within 60 minutes. The importance of drawing up such standards is that they should be realisable and, importantly, can be audited. Indeed, potential purchasers may require evidence that regular audit of the service is undertaken. Such audit is usually performed in conjunction with users, who benefit from the information gained. Such a partnership allows the service to grow with the demands placed upon it and to be flexible in its delivery. Many laboratories are taking part in this process, which is all part of Continual Quality Improvement, and is vital if laboratories are to continue to provide a high-quality service. Again, purchasers may wish to have information on such processes in provider laboratories.

MARKETING

It is no longer sufficient for laboratories providing a clinical service to remain as passive players in the new market-place with GPs. Laboratories must actively promote themselves in terms of the service provided and must target their services appropriately. Marketing may be defined as identifying, anticipating and satisfying client needs profitably. Although the profit element is not presently permitted in the public sector, many laboratories would define profitable as staying in business or surviving.

There is little doubt that the most successful laboratories, especially in terms of dialogue with GPs, have good relationships with their users, which have taken time to establish and can only be set up by liaison and good communication. This is the essence of good marketing and it is vital that laboratory staff meet their major users on a regular basis. In this way, defects in the service, which may not be formally articulated clearly as complaints, can be addressed and GPs can see that the laboratories are serious about listening and attending to problems effectively.

Similarly, laboratories can find out about new services that GPs are planning and respond appropriately while GPs can learn about new tests and developments in the service generally. Laboratories have a central role in organising such meetings and all opportunities must be taken e.g., informal lunch-time meetings, case conferences, tutorials etc.

CONTRACTS

GPs will either have contracts placed directly with a hospital laboratory (as fundholders) or will have contracts via the District Health Authority, which negotiates agreements on behalf of non-fundholding GPs. Initially, contracts have been of a block contract type, whereby a batch of services is purchased *in toto* from the hospital laboratory. Many of the early contracts did not realistically reflect true costs and were very approximate. Additionally, they did not allow for variation in requesting and were thus insensitive. Newer contracts are more likely to be of a cost and volume type and to reflect more closely market variations. Contracts may vary enormously but for GPs to have confidence in them, they should specify many of the factors mentioned above e.g., transport, phlebotomy, turnaround time, standards and audit. As experience grows in this area, the contracts will become much better defined. Figure 2.7 illustrates an example of a contract (headings only).

Service Agreement for Pathology Laboratory Services

between

Meadsmere Practice and City Hospital

Objectives

Services covered (& exclusions) - including phlebotomy if relevant

Volume and mix

Price and tolerance e.g., +/- 10% of estimated volume

Billing and payment

Communication arrangements

      - request forms

      - clinically urgent arrangements phone / fax

      - courier

Quality standards

Variation of service - renegotiation, arbitration, non-performance.

Figure 2.7   **Service agreement for pathology laboratory services**

PROVIDERS OF THE SERVICE

The following may provide a laboratory service:

- local hospital

- private laboratory (either stand-alone or within private hospital)

- distant factory laboratories

- near-patient facility.

Figure 2.8   Providers of service

Apart from the cost, which is being increasingly used by some as the sole criterion of where to place a contract, a number of other factors must be considered in making a decision. Many of these factors have been described in the preceding sections and include: phlebotomy, transport and also an interactive service including interpretive help. GPs, in common with all purchasers of services, must carefully determine their needs before choosing a particular provider.

NEAR-PATIENT TESTING

Near-patient testing has been around under other names for many years e.g., the dipstick for urine glucose, which of course is testing near the patient. Although the last decade has seen the burgeoning of analysers which can be used in GP practices, we must not forget the value of dipstick tests appropriately used as a contribution to patient care. Dipstick tests have increased in scope and now include indicators of microbiological infection as well as the traditional estimations.

The enormous increase in near-patient testing procedures, other than dipsticks which was said by many to herald the decline of hospital laboratories, has now plateaued and is probably falling. This has nothing to do with the potential quality of analyses possible with such instruments when used properly, but all to do with the practicality, the clinical usefulness and the cost. Many instruments were placed in surgeries with little attention to the long-term needs of training, maintenance, quality control, documentation and safety. Indeed, instruments may have had a capital value which was immediately written off, without the GP being aware of the future revenue consequences i.e., the cost of running the instrument. Not surprisingly, some GPs became disenchanted with the provision of, say, on-site cholesterol measurements and have reverted back to using the local laboratory. Some of this may be due to the time required to perform the test and the inconvenience in doing so and also the uncertain clinical relevance of performing a test immediately, which additionally may have an influence on allowing 'time to think'.

However, there is a place for near-patient testing and a nationally agreed set of guidelines has been established. Figure 2.9 is a summary version of the near-patient testing guidelines (headings only).

1. **Analyses and Equipment**
- What are you going to measure?
- Which equipment is most suitable for your purpose?
- What are the likely costs?

2. **Looking After The Equipment**
- How will you look after the equipment?
- What will you do when the equipment does not work?

3. **Health and Safety**
- Will you be able to initiate and maintain the required health & safety procedures?

4. **Personnel Requirements**
- What particular skills will they need?
- How will the staff be trained?

5. **Quality Assurance**
- Can you trust your reports?
- How will the results be recorded?

6. **Interpretation of Results**
- Who will be responsible for the interpretation of results?
- Who should supply additional expert help with interpretation?

Figure 2.9   Near patient testing guidelines

For further details refer to Appendix I.

FURTHER READING

NHS Executive, Strategic Review of Pathology Services. London: HMSO, 1995.

Hobbs R. Near patient testing in primary care. BMJ 1996; 312: 263-264.

Millman A, Lee N, Brooke A. Computers in General Practice – I. BMJ 1995; 311; 800 – 802.

Chapter 3

The Interpretation of Laboratory Data

William Marshall

INTRODUCTION

Doctors request laboratory tests for various reasons, but in every case the request is, or should be, framed to answer a particular question. In order that the question can be answered, it is clearly essential that the appropriate test is requested and that the result can be relied on.

This chapter examines some of the uses of laboratory tests, and how they should be interpreted. We also consider some of the potential sources of error.

THE USES OF LABORATORY TESTS

The uses of laboratory tests are summarized in Figure 3.1

- to provide information to support (or refute) a clinical diagnosis

- to extend a clinical diagnosis by providing information about causation

- to indicate the presence of complications, including complications of treatment

- to provide prognostic information

- to monitor the progress of a condition (either its natural history or the response to treatment)

- to detect sub-clinical disease ('screening').

Figure 3.1   Uses of laboratory tests

Other, more specialised uses, include the stratification of patients for the purpose of drug trials, the detection of drug toxicity in trials, etc. These latter uses are not discussed in this book.

THE QUALITY OF LABORATORY DATA

In the laboratory, considerable care is taken to ensure that appropriate procedures for sample handling, documentation and analysis are adhered to in order to maximize the accuracy and precision of the results. (**Accuracy** is an indication of how near the result is to the correct value; **precision** is an indication of how reproducible the result is, see Figure 3.2.) All laboratories use rigorous internal quality control procedures, involving, for example, the repeated analysis of samples of known composition; they also participate in external quality assurance schemes, where samples of unknown composition are tested and the results compared with those from other laboratories.

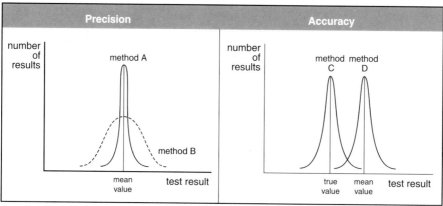

Figure 3.2 Precision and accuracy of laboratory tests.
Precision is a measure of reproducibility, accuracy of the nearness of a measured value to the actual value. The graphs show the distribution of values for measurements of the same analyte by different methods. Methods A and B are equally accurate but A is more precise than method B (less scatter about mean); methods C and D have equal precision, but C is more accurate.

The introduction of national schemes for laboratory accreditation should further enhance the quality of the results that laboratories produce, since the granting of accreditation requires adherence to a range of quality related standards (see Chapter 2).

There are, however, a number of factors which can influence the results of laboratory tests, over which the laboratory may have no direct control. These are divided into pre-analytical and post-analytical factors. Examples of these are shown in Figure 3.3.

Such matters are addressed in the users' handbooks produced by laboratories. Users hoping to obtain a good service from their local laboratory should make use of this handbook, and not hesitate to telephone the laboratory if they require advice before collecting a sample or requesting a particular test. It is frustrating and wasteful for the doctor, laboratory staff and patient if a test cannot be performed because a sample was incorrectly collected, or if the result cannot be found because the sample was incorrectly labelled.

Pre-analytical factors

- the collection of the correct sample, under appropriate conditions

- appropriate preservation and handling

- rapid transport to the laboratory

- secure indentification

Post-analytical factors

- calculation error

- transmission error

- transcription error

Figure 3.3   Pre- and post-analytical factors affecting the results of laboratory tests

Guidance to sample requirements for the more frequently requested laboratory tests is given where the test is discussed (see Chapter 7).

THE INTERPRETATION OF LABORATORY DATA

It is important that the doctor should appreciate the potential benefits and limitations of individual tests in the context in which they are used. Laboratories offer a formidable and ever-growing repertoire of tests and individual practitioners are only likely to become familiar with those that they use frequently. It is always prudent to seek the advice of the laboratory when considering laboratory tests in relation to an unusual or complex clinical problem, or when an unfamiliar test seems appropriate in the clinical context.

In general, the results of laboratory tests, particularly if they are quantitative, that is, their results are expressed numerically, can give rise to one or both of two questions:

- Is the result indicative of health or disease, and if of disease, is it diagnostic of a condition?

- Is the result different from one obtained previously, and if so, is it clinically significant?

It may be noted that, while high accuracy and precision are always desirable, accuracy (see above) is paramount when tests are performed primarily for diagnosis while precision is paramount when patients are being monitored by serial testing.

Similar questions can be asked in relation to qualitative results (for example, is there any evidence of malignancy in a cytological smear?) but while it is generally accepted that there may be a place for an individual opinion in this context, the fact that many laboratory data are quantitative tends to obscure the undoubted fact that even with the results of the highest quality, there may be some uncertainty as to their interpretation.

The apparent simplicity of these questions in relation to quantitative data belies their complexity. An understanding of the principles that govern their answering is essential to the interpretation, and thus to the rational use, of laboratory data.

WHAT IS NORMAL?

'Normal' is a word with several distinct meanings and shades of meaning. These include: 'regular', 'acceptable', 'usual', 'conforming to a type' and 'healthy'. 'Normal' also has different precise meanings in science (as in, for example, a normal solution) and in mathematics. It is synonymous with 'Gaussian', describing the distribution of a particular variable in a population such that this conforms to the familiar bell-shaped symmetrical distribution about a mean (Figure 3.4).

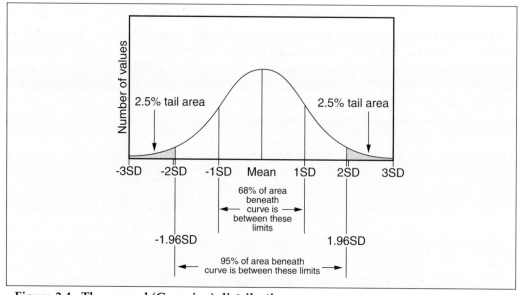

Figure 3.4   The normal (Gaussian) distribution.
Measured values are distributed symmetrically about the mean. The normal range encompasses values falling between two standard deviations below and two standard deviations above the mean, and includes approximately 95% of all values.

If a variable has a Gaussian distribution, the range of values from two standard deviations less than the mean to two standard deviations greater than the mean encompasses 95% of the total. This range is called the 'normal range', and is widely used as a standard against which to compare observational data, to provide an indication of how such data relate to the same measurement made in a large population. The 'population' in the context of the interpretation of laboratory data means a group of comparable, healthy individuals. Comparability is important. Like must be compared with like, so that if the distribution of a variable depends on e.g., age, sex, etc., the observed value should be evaluated against the normal range for a population of the same age, sex, etc.

Two major problems arise from the use of the term 'normal range', and have led to attempts by laboratory personnel (rarely adopted by clinicians) to introduce alternative terms.

The first is that, by definition, the normal range encompasses only 95% of values in the normal population. This means that a value lying outside the range could still be observed in the population and may therefore not be 'abnormal' (although clearly the likelihood of its being so will increase, the further displaced from the extremes of the range it is). Second, 'normal' as defined scientifically may not be equivalent to the less precise meanings given above, that is, healthy, usual, or acceptable.

This second point is well illustrated by considering the significance of plasma cholesterol measurements. Elevated cholesterol concentrations are a major risk factor for the development of coronary heart disease. The 'normal range' for cholesterol, as derived from measurements on healthy adults, is approximately 3.5-6.7mmol/L. However, it is established that the risk of coronary heart disease increases with increasing cholesterol concentrations even within this range, such that, for example, the risk is doubled between cholesterols of 5.2mmol/L and 6.7mmol/L. Furthermore, although the gradient of the risk/concentration line becomes very shallow at cholesterol concentrations below 5.2mmol/L, it never entirely flattens out (Figure 3.5).

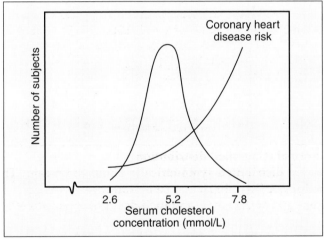

Figure 3.5 Serum cholesterol concentrations in healthy individuals and the risk of coronary heart disease. The risk of coronary heart disease increases with increasing cholesterol concentration even within the range found in healthy individuals. Approximately one third of the adult population have values greater than the generally accepted highest desirable cholesterol concentration. Note also that cholesterol concentrations do not have a Gaussian distribution: there is a skew towards higher values.

There is therefore a contradiction between the precise meaning of 'normal' in the term 'normal range' and that of 'healthy' or 'acceptable' in the context of plasma cholesterol concentration. It is noteworthy that many laboratories now quote 'ideal' or 'desirable' ranges for plasma cholesterol concentration although it should be appreciated that these are dependent on the clinical circumstances.

Not all biological variables have a Gaussian distribution in a healthy population, but, according to the nature of the distribution, it is usually possible mathematically to transform the data to fit a Gaussian distribution so that the same principles can be applied.

This discussion may seem to be largely semantic, but patients, and doctors, often ask if a result is normal; they may be misled if they are using the word in a different context to the laboratory staff.

For such reasons, it has been recommended that the term 'normal range' be abandoned. Instead, it is suggested that results should be compared with those from a 'reference population' in whom upper and lower 'reference limits' encompass a 'reference interval'. The term 'reference', being free of any connotations of health or acceptability, should lead to more objective interpretation of laboratory data, but it has not yet become widely used outside laboratories. In fact, most reference intervals are numerically based on the former normal ranges, so that the term 'reference' appears somewhat artificial.

A potential advantage of the use of reference limits is that, being free of connotations of health or acceptability, such intervals could be determined for pathological conditions, allowing a result to be compared not only with the range of values expected in health but also with that characteristic of a given disease.

However, reference intervals are not generally available for diseases although there is no intrinsic reason why they should not be. Indeed, given knowledge of the distribution and range of values for a particular test in health and disease, it would be possible to ascribe a probability to any observed value having occurred in either a healthy or diseased individual. The specificities of tests for disease varies. Thus the erythrocyte sedimentation rate (ESR) is non-specific, being increased in many acute and chronic illnesses, while abnormalities of plasma calcium concentration (for example) occur in a relatively small number of conditions.

In practice, what matters is whether a given test result provides the answer to the question that prompted the test request. Test requests, and thus results, fall into two general categories: ones that are being made for the first time in a patient (e.g., for screening or diagnosis), and those that are being repeated (e.g., for monitoring). In the first instance, the result must be compared with what is expected; in the second, it can be compared with a previous result, to see if a significant change has occurred.

For most laboratory tests, there is an overlap between the values characteristic of health and those found in disease. Common sense tells us that the more 'abnormal' a result is (barring error), the more likely it is to represent a pathological process. But given that, by definition, 5% of healthy individuals will have results outside the limits of the range encompassed by two standard deviations either side of the mean, a result outside this range may not be exceptional for that individual.

Greater diagnostic accuracy is often provided by measuring two or more relevant variables (as in the case of hypothyroidism, see below), but the more tests that are performed, the more likely it is that one will show a result outside the reference interval which is not of pathological significance.

THE USE OF LABORATORY TESTS FOR DIAGNOSIS

Two general problems impede the use of laboratory tests for diagnosis. First, and particularly with quantitative biochemical and haematological tests, there is usually an overlap between the results of a test that can occur in healthy individuals and those with disease (that is, the reference ranges overlap, see Figure 3.6). Thus individuals with early non-insulin dependent diabetes may have elevated blood glucose concentrations only after meals, but have fasting values within the reference range for healthy individuals. Similarly, impaired renal function may not cause the plasma creatinine to be elevated until the glomerular filtration rate has fallen to one half of normal (Figure 3.7).

Second, many laboratory tests are not specific for individual diseases. A clinical suspicion of anaemia may prompt measurement of the haemoglobin. A low value confirms the diagnosis by definition but can be the result of numerous pathological processes which cause anaemia. However, the additional demonstration of hypochromasia and microcytosis suggests that anaemia may be due to iron deficiency; this would be confirmed by the demonstration of low marrow iron stores, but even then, any of a number of possible causes, e.g., dietary deficiency, malabsorption and excessive loss could be responsible. To take another example, a high plasma free thyroxine concentration is characteristic of (though not specific to) hyperthyroidism; if the plasma concentration of thyroid stimulating hormone (TSH) is low, this supports the diagnosis and suggests primary thyroid disease as the cause, but neither test, alone or in combination, indicates the cause of this abnormality, e.g., Graves' disease, solitary adenoma, etc.

SCREENING FOR DISEASE

The overlap between test values seen in health and disease is of particular relevance to the practice of so called biochemical and haematological screening, that is, performing a battery of tests in individuals with no clinical evidence of a particular disease whose presence might be indicated by an abnormal result in one or more of the tests.

If, say, measurements of ten independent biochemical variables were made (independent meaning that the cause of an abnormality in one would not tend to cause another to be abnormal), the probability that at least one would be outside the reference interval would be 0.95^{10} (0.95, or 1 in 20, being the probability of a single result falling outside this range). This is equal to approximately 0.6. Thus a little over one out of every two sets of ten tests

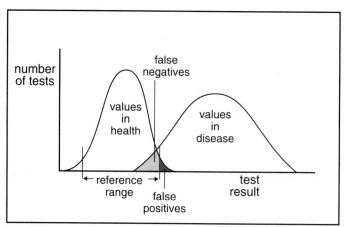

Figure 3.6 Distribution of results of a biochemical test in groups of individuals with and without disease.

The distribution of values is continuous, so that some individuals with disease have normal values and some healthy individuals have values more characteristic of disease. The test gives false positive results (high value, no disease) and false negative results (normal value, disease present).

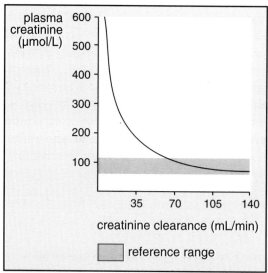

Figure 3.7 Plasma creatinine concentration and creatinine clearance (a measure of the glomerular filtration rate, GFR).

Because clearance is determined by the reciprocal of plasma creatinine concentration (1/[creatinine]), a significant decrease in GFR may occur before the plasma creatinine concentration increases beyond the reference range.

performed in a group of healthy people would be expected to show one result outside the reference interval.

The more tests performed, the greater the likelihood of such a result. In general, however, this is not a practical problem, for such results are usually only slightly outside the reference interval and informed judgment will lead to the 'abnormality' being appropriately judged as of no significance. If the significance is uncertain, the test can be repeated or, better, an alternative test, which provides similar information, performed. If a screening test throws up a clearly abnormal result (and by definition it will be in the absence of a related clinical abnormality), the adage that it is the patient, not the test result, that should be treated, still holds good. While isolated abnormalities in test results must not be ignored, they should not prompt treatment without confirmation and, if necessary, further investigation.

For laboratory tests used in screening for disease, in which there is a continuum of results characteristic of health and disease, cut-off values must be defined to separate those judged at low risk of having the condition, and those requiring further investigation. This will often be the upper (or lower) reference limit, but the value chosen should be that which does the job required of it — that is, sorts those tested into appropriate categories, essentially into groups requiring and not requiring further investigation.

The cut-off chosen will depend on what is required of the test. If it is vital to detect all individuals with a disease the cut-off should be set lower than the lower limit seen in disease. Such an approach will succeed in detecting affected individuals, but at the expense of falsely categorizing a number of healthy people, who may be subjected to unnecessary further investigation before they are proved to be free of the disease. On the other hand, if the limit is set higher, some individuals with disease will be mis-classified, although fewer healthy people will be (see Figure 3.8). To be technical, setting the cut-off low makes the test highly *sensitive* (positive in the presence of disease) but not very *specific* (negative in health); setting it high has the reverse effect — it is *less sensitive* (not all with disease are identified), but *more specific* (fewer healthy people are mis-classified). Such considerations are of particular importance in screening newborn infants for inherited metabolic disease, in antenatal screening and in screening for cancer, where the consequences of a wrong diagnosis may be catastrophic.

These concepts of sensitivity and specificity are becoming more frequently used in assessments of the value of laboratory tests, although they remain generally poorly understood. Their calculation is shown in Figure 3.9.

If the prevalence of a condition in the population screened is known, *predictive values* can be calculated, which indicate the probability that a given test result (positive or negative) correctly assigns the patient to the health or disease category. Such information can be used to determine management. Thus there is a general consensus that if a man is found to have a prostate-specific antigen concentration exceeding $10\mu g/L$, the probability of his having prostatic cancer is sufficiently great for him to require urgent urological assessment. If the concentration is below $10\mu g/L$, the likelihood of cancer, and the urgency, is less.

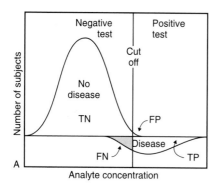

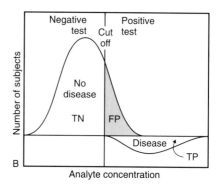

Figure 3.8 Sensitivity and specificity.
When the ranges of results for a test that occur in health and disease overlap, a cut-off
value may be applied to determine whether a result is regarded as positive (for the
disease) or negative. Setting a high cut-off value (A) minimises the number of false
positives and maximises the specificity but the number of false negatives increases,
reducing the sensitivity. Setting a lower cut-off value (B) has the opposite effect.

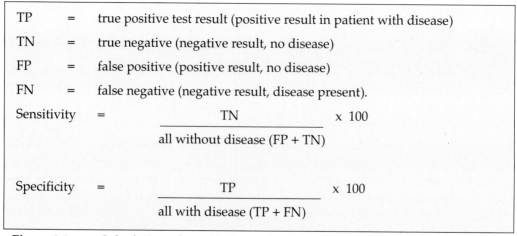

Figure 3.9   Calculation of specificity and sensitivity of a test

MONITORING AND FOLLOW-UP

When laboratory data are used for this purpose, the result of a test can be compared with one done previously. Thus a repeat haemoglobin measurement will indicate whether there has been a response to a course of iron tablets, a repeat cholesterol to dietary counselling, a repeat glycated haemoglobin to an increase in oral hypoglycaemics, etc.

But a change in the result of a test may not be of clinical significance. Whether a change is of significance will depend on the circumstances. For example, even a minor decrease in the glycated haemoglobin may be worth achieving in a young, insulin-dependent diabetic patient (improved control now being established as being linked to a decreased risk of long term complications), but will be of less importance for an elderly diabetic patient whose main concern will be freedom from acute symptoms.

But before a change can be judged to be clinically significant, account must be taken of natural, biological variation, and of analytical variation. No quantitative analytical test is completely precise (gives exactly the same result each time it is performed on a given specimen), despite the efforts that laboratory staff make to minimize imprecision. Furthermore, even if it were, repeated performance of the same test on the same individual under the same conditions over a period of time would not produce the same result time after time. It would produce a set of similar results, clustering around a mean. Anyone who uses bathroom scales regularly should have first-hand experience of these principles.

Both analytical and biological variation can be measured. They can be combined to give an indication of the extent of any change that is 'real' — that is, unlikely to be due to chance (although not necessarily of clinical significance). It is not necessary to reproduce the calculation here, but the 'critical value' of a test indicates the extent of change which is likely to be 'real' at any level of probability. Critical values ($p<0.05$, that is, a probability of less than 1 in 20 of the observed change being due to chance variation) for some frequently performed tests are shown in Figure 3.10.

Such data are worthy of wide dissemination. All too frequently one sees a clinical decision being made on the basis of a change which is unlikely to be significant. The opposite — failure to react to significant change — also occurs. Neither should occur, and it is a responsibility of the laboratory staff to advise users of their service in this area, for example by providing interpretative reports or by publishing lists of critical differences.

Analyte	Level	Units	Change Absolute	%
Sodium	140	mmol/L	6	4
Potassium	4.2	mmol/L	0.6	14
Calcium (total)	2.4	mmol/L	0.19	8
Magnesium	1.0	mmol/L	0.4	40
Phosphate	1.2	mmol/L	0.3	25
Bicarbonate	26	mmol/L	4	15
Urea	5.0	mmol/L	2.1	43
Creatinine	60	μmol/L	21	35
Urate	0.26	mmol/L	0.07	3
Glucose	4.6	mmol/L	1.6	35
Bilirubin (total)	10	mmol/L	10	100
Cholesterol	5.8	mmol/L	1.6	27
Triglycerides	1.2	mmol/L	0.9	75
Total protein	75	g/L	6	8
Albumin	40	g/L	5	13
ALP	60	U/L	22	37
AST	20	U/L	13	65
γGT	40	U/L	40	100

Figure 3.10   Examples of critical changes

Based on data from Fraser CG. Interpretation of clinical laboratory data. Blackwell Scientific Publications, 1986

FURTHER READING

Marshall WJ. Clinical Chemistry (3rd edition). London: Mosby, 1995.

Fraser CG. Interpretation of clinical chemistry laboratory data. Oxford: Blackwell Scientific Publications, 1986.

Morris HA. Strategies for interpretation of clincial laboratory data. Clin Biochem Rev 1991; 12: 34-37.

Fraser CG, Fogarty Y. Interpreting laboratory results. BMJ. 1989; 298: 1659-1660.

Chapter 4

Histopathology and Cytopathology

Stephen Humphreys & Romil Saxena

Histopathology deals with tissue diagnosis of disease whereas cytopathology is diagnosis based on the analysis of individual cells which have either been shed from mucosal surfaces (exfoliative cytology) or aspirated from a lesion by a fine needle (Fine Needle Aspiration Cytology [FNAC]). Dealing with complete tissue histopathological examination allows appreciation of architectural patterns, maturational details and tissue relationships and offers a distinct advantage over cytopathological examination, although fine needle aspirates may sometimes include larger fragments of tissue which are in effect microbiopsies. Obtaining adequate FNAC specimens is a challenging technique and success largely depends on the expertise and experience of the operator, it is therefore unlikely to achieve wide usage in primary care where insufficient numbers will be performed to allow such experience to be gained.

In a typical histo/cytopathology laboratory, endoscopic gastrointestinal, bronchoscopic and colposcopic biopsies, skin biopsies and cervical cytology smears comprise the majority of specimens received. The histopathologist also deals with all resection specimens from major operations and plays a key role in the diagnostic process. In this chapter, we will largely confine the discussion to dermatopathology and cervical cytology as these are by far the most common types of specimen to reach the histopathology laboratory from the general practitioner.

SKIN BIOPSY

Skin biopsies may be obtained in one of four ways.

1. The shave biopsy, as the name suggests, shaves off the epidermis and superficial dermis. The technique affords good cosmesis and is often used to remove disfiguring lesions on the face. Intradermal nevi can be effectively dealt with in this way.

2. The excision biopsy removes the skin lesion, usually an elliptical piece of skin with a circumferential margin of normal skin and includes the deep dermis and superficial subcutaneous tissue. Some studies have shown that there is a higher incidence of incomplete excision of lesions emanating from the GPs' surgeries and this has been related to a more frequent failure

to suspect malignancy by the GP versus the dermatologist.

3. The punch biopsy samples the epidermis, dermis and the superficial subcutaneous tissue. It measures between 2-5mm in diameter.

4. The incisional biopsy samples one half or one edge of a skin lesion with the adjacent uninvolved skin.

The punch biopsy and incisional skin biopsy are diagnostic biopsies and do not aim to remove the lesion.

Some lesions, such as seborrhoeic keratoses, are amenable to curettage but the fragmented nature of the specimen obtained renders histological interpretation difficult and therefore this technique should be used with caution when the diagnosis is really uncertain clinically. It is perhaps superfluous to stress the importance of submitting all tissue removed from the patient for histological analysis as even the most carefully considered clinical diagnosis may be incorrect. There are indeed many reports in the literature of malignancy in lesions described clinically as sebaceous cysts.

Most non-neoplastic skin diseases are dynamic, evolving over a period of time and diagnostic features might only be seen at one point of their evolution. Thus it is necessary to biopsy either the most classical or an early lesion rather than one complicated by secondary features. Such skin biopsies are rarely submitted from the GPs' surgeries as diagnostic skin biopsies have usually remained the domain of dermatologists, except for those GPs with a special interest.

TISSUE FIXATION

Tissues should be fixed immediately to preserve cellular detail and prevent degradation of cellular components. Fixation also hardens tissue and this is necessary for the subsequent cutting of sections for microscopy. Formalin is the best all-purpose fixative for routine diagnosis and appropriate for fixation of skin biopsies. Formalin is a solution in water of 40% formaldehyde gas by weight. It is used as a 10% solution in water buffered with sodium phosphate to prevent formation of formic acid which turns the solution acidic and is not conducive to proper fixation. It should be noted that tissue should be placed immediately into fixative and requires about 10 times its own volume for proper fixation. On no account should a biopsy be crammed into a pot which is inadequate in size.

Various other fixatives are available, some of which may be advantageous for demonstration of certain specific components. Some circumstances e.g., techniques being employed in molecular biology for both research and diagnosis, require fresh tissue which needs to be rapidly transported to the laboratory in dry ice. Fresh, unfixed tissue is also required for immunofluorescence which is used for diagnosis of non-infectious vesiculobullous diseases and autoimmune diseases like systemic lupus erythematosus (SLE). Such investigations are unlikely to be required by the general practitioner but, before obtaining a specimen biopsy for any specialised investigation, advice should be obtained from the laboratory regarding optimal handling and transport. It cannot be stressed too highly that adequate fixation is essential to the diagnostic process and poorly fixed specimens are often difficult if not impossible to interpret. Fortunately the days of biopsies reaching the laboratory in jam jars containing the most convenient spirit to hand, e.g., whisky, appear to be over.

DESPATCH TO THE LABORATORY

The specimen container should be labelled with the patient's name, sex, date of birth and the nature of the specimen. The same particulars should be entered on the request form. It is extremely important to provide full clinical information. Interpretation of skin biopsies is one of the most difficult areas in tissue diagnosis and is almost impossible without clinical information. The pathologist recognises a pattern of histological features which he must then correlate with clinical details like age, sex, site, distribution and gross appearance of lesions to arrive at an accurate, definitive diagnosis. The appearances of the biopsy reflects a relatively limited set of pathobiological processes and therefore there is often overlap in the histological appearances of different conditions. Under these circumstances, full clinical information can often help to separate them.

DESCRIPTION OF THE COMMON SKIN LESIONS

There follows a brief description of some of the more common lesions which find their way from primary care to the histopathology laboratory.

It is not intended to be a comprehensive dermatopathological survey but merely to act as a source of information and glossary of terms when confronted with the report. If there is anything contained in the report which is not understood or does not appear to make sense, speak personally to the pathologist. Most histopathologists will in fact telephone the general practitioner if the biopsy yields a surprising or unusual lesion.

ACTINIC KERATOSIS

Actinic keratosis, also known as solar keratosis, is associated with sun exposure and is extremely common (Figure 4.1). It occurs particularly on the head and neck region. Atypia of the basal layer of the epidermis is the hallmark of actinic keratosis along with evidence of actinic damage to the dermal collagen which shows increased staining and fragmentation due to the effects of ultraviolet light. Although actinic keratosis is considered to be a premalignant lesion, the incidence of progression to squamous carcinoma is actually less than 1%. However their presence serves to alert one to the fact that this individual is sun-damaged and may develop other sun related problems in the future.

Pathologists may qualify actinic keratosis as hyperkeratotic, atrophic, acantholytic, lichenoid, epidermolytic or spreading pigmented actinic keratosis. These are histological variants with no biologic significance.

BOWEN'S DISEASE AND CARCINOMA-IN-SITU

Bowen's disease is a term used synonymously with squamous carcinoma-in-situ. Histologically, the term carcinoma-in-situ is used for full thickness dysplasia of any epithelium. Biologically, it denotes a pre-invasive lesion. Carcinoma-in-situ of the skin does not invariably lead to invasive cancer and in fact, invasion occurs only rarely. Bowen's disease, erythroplasia of Queyrat (affecting the glans penis), bowenoid papulosis and bowenoid actinic keratosis are generally included in the group comprising carcinoma-in-situ. Bowen's disease presents clinically as an erythematous plaque on the lower abdomen, buttocks, or most commonly the lower legs (Figure 4.2). Histologically, there is full thickness dysplasia but the actual progression to invasive carcinoma is rare (about 2.5%). When a histologically similar lesion appears on the glans penis or the vulva or mucous membranes, the potential for invasion is higher. Bowenoid papulosis is an interesting member of this group that has caused a lot of confusion. Bowenoid papulosis appears as groups of pigmented papules in the ano-genital regions of young adults. Histologically, there is full thickness dysplasia but the lesions are known to regress and progression to invasive disease is extremely rare. The lesion is caused by human papilloma virus (HPV), usually type 16.

BASAL CELL CARCINOMA

Basal cell carcinoma is an extremely common tumour that occurs on sun-exposed sites (Figure 4.3). A true basal cell carcinoma never metastasizes and most of these tumours are completely cured by curettage. The tumour is composed of downgrowth of cells resembling the basal cells of the epidermis.

The pathology report may sometimes describe variants of basal cell carcinoma; only two of these have any biologic significance. Morphea-like type of basal cell carcinoma is deeply infiltrative, difficult to excise completely and prone to recurrence. If suspected, the patient is best referred for specialist excision. The superficial or multicentric variant consists of small tumour nodules that do not extend beyond the superficial dermis. This type is often ill-defined clinically and may be incompletely excised leading to the risk of local recurrence.

SQUAMOUS CELL CARCINOMA AND KERATOACANTHOMA

Squamous cell carcinoma is a relatively common lesion, most are actinically induced and have a relatively benign clinical course (Figure 4.4); metastasis can occur but is uncommon. The risk of recurrence is doubled, and that of metastases trebled, in tumours measuring 2 cm or more.

Keratoacanthoma is a curious lesion which mimics a squamous cell carcinoma, both clinically and histologically. The patient presents with a keratotic nodule that grows at an alarming rate over a 6 - 8 week period. Histologically, there is a central crater filled with keratin and surrounded by keratinocytic proliferation which is difficult and sometimes impossible to distinguish from a squamous cell carcinoma. The classical evolution of the nodule is an important clue to the diagnosis because after the rapid growth phase, the lesion appears to slow down and then regress. Most lesions tend to be excised during the rapid growth phase.

VERRUCA VULGARIS

The common wart is occasionally excised for cosmetic reasons or because of uncertain diagnosis (Figure 4.5). Excision is not the optimal treatment, as the recurrence rate is much higher after excision than cryotherapy. They are caused by the human papilloma virus which induces squamous proliferation. HPV types 2, 4 and 7 are responsible for verruca vulgaris and 1 and 2 for plantar warts. Histopathological diagnosis of active lesions is straightforward due to distinctive cytopathic changes with enlarged keratohyaline granules in the granular layer of the epidermis. These features may be absent in older lesions and these may receive a descriptive report such as "warty keratosis".

SEBORRHOEIC KERATOSIS/ BASAL CELL PAPILLOMA

Seborrhoeic keratosis is a very common lesion appearing on the trunk and face of middle aged people as small, sharply demarcated, verrucous or keratotic papules that look as if they have been stuck on the surface of the skin (Figure 4.6). Occasionally, they are pedunculated, appearing as a soft fibroma. Histologically, an exophytic epidermal proliferation of small keratinocytic cells with interspersed horn cysts is seen. The term basal cell papilloma should not be confused with basal cell carcinoma.

FIBROUS PAPULE OF THE FACE

Fibrous papule of the face or nose occurs as a small, solitary, firm, dome-shaped lesion not exceeding 0.5 cm in diameter on the nose of adults. The lesion has been variously regarded as an angiofibroma, a perifollicular fibroma and an involuting nevus. Histologically, the lesions show stellate cells that are considered to be fibroblasts by some and melanocytes by others. Some cases show prominent blood vessels, others show perifollicular fibrosis. In any case, the lesion is benign.

DERMATOFIBROMA

Dermatofibroma is a very common lesion that occurs most often on the extremities in adult life as a firm, slightly raised nodule which often becomes pigmented (Figure 4.7). The dermatofibroma is a benign tumour of fibroblasts in which spindle cells are arranged from a central point in a whorl like fashion. The spindle cells blend impercetibly into the collagen of the adjacent dermis.

MOLLUSCUM CONTAGIOSUM

Molluscum contagiosum is caused by a pox virus with characteristic clinical and pathological features. The lesion occurs as small, waxy 2 - 4 mm papules with an umbilicated center (Figure 4.8). Histologically, the epidermis assumes a lobulated appearance and the keratinocytes contain prominent eosinophilic inclusions occupying and enlarging the nucleus.

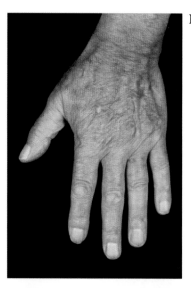

Fig.4.1 Actinic keratosis: Small firm hyperkeratotic lesions on a sun exposed site (dorsum of the hand)

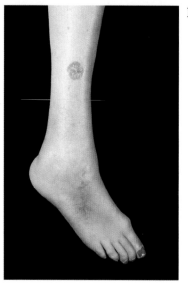

Fig.4.2 Bowen's disease: A solitary plaque of red scaly skin, typically on the lower leg of an elderly female

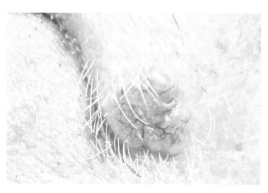

Fig.4.3 Basal cell carcinoma: A translucent nodule with prominent telangiectasia occuring in the nasolabial fold. This is the cystic variant of a BCC

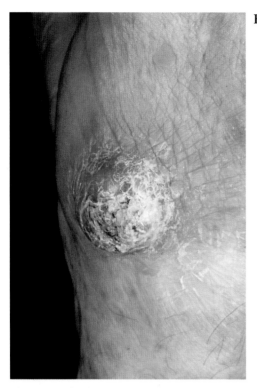

Fig.4.4 Squamous cell carcinoma: A large rapidly growing, infiltrative nodule arising on sun-damaged skin

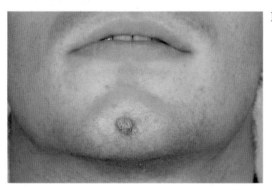

Fig.4.5 Viral wart: Small firm hyperkeratotic papules which on the face often have a filiform surface

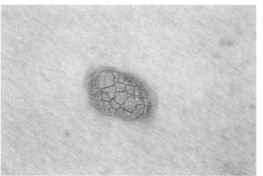

Fig.4.6 Seborrhoeic keratosis: A crusty pigmented lesion with well-circumscribed margins and a fissured, coarse greasy surface

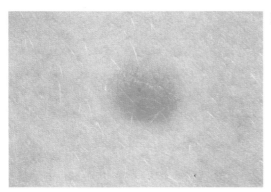

Fig.4.7 Dermatofibroma: A firm, smooth and well-circumscribed, small papule within the dermis, which may develop a pigmented rim with age

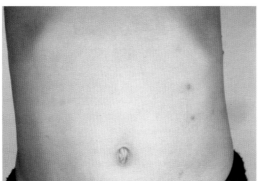

Fig.4.8 Mollusca contagiosum: These small pearly viral papules are very common in children, in whom spontananeous resolution is the norm. Larger, solitary lesions in adults may be amenable to curretage

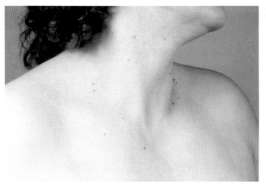

Fig.4.9 Fibroepithelial polyp: Numerous small flesh-coloured skin tags around the collar line

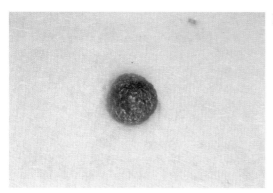

Fig.4.10 Benign compound nevus: A well-circumscribed pigmented lesion, evenly coloured throughout

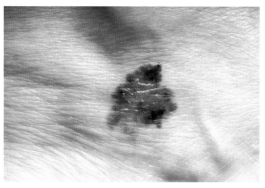

Fig.4.11 Cellular nevi: flesh-coloured domed lesions occuring particularly on the face. They are very amenable to shave biopsy

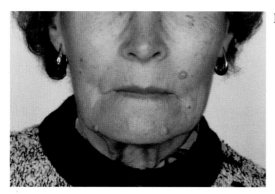

Fig.4.12 Malignant melanoma: This superficial spreading melanoma has been growing recently and the lesion has an irregular margin and variable pigmentation within

FIBROEPITHELIAL POLYP

The fibroepithelial polyp or skin tag is perhaps the commonest skin lesion removed for cosmetic reasons. Skin tags can occur as single or multiple lesions with a smooth, filiform or furrowed surface (Figure 4.9). Histologically, the skin tag is covered by acanthotic, hyperkeratotic epidermis with papillomatosis and consists of a fibrous core which sometimes contains nevus cells. A few skin tags contain mature fat cells and are believed to arise from involuted nevi.

MELANOCYTIC LESIONS

The benign acquired nevus is the most common melanocytic lesion encountered in the general population and is excised either for cosmetic reasons or because it is feared to be malignant. The benign nevus goes through an orderly process of evolution in its natural history and the histology and clinical appearance reflect these changes. The lesion begins as a deeply pigmented, well circumscribed, slightly pigmented papule, usually less than 0.6 cm in diameter (Figure 4.10). Histologically, this corresponds to the junctional nevus in which nests of benign melanocytes are found at the dermal-epidermal junction. Nests of nevus cells next appear in the dermis in addition to the epidermal-dermal junction. This is the compound nevus which now appears less pigmented and dome-shaped. The compound nevus evolves into the intradermal nevus as the junctional component disappears and the nevus cells are completely within the dermis. This lesion is dome-shaped and the colour of normal skin (Figure 4.11). Over many years, most nevi tend to involute and this may be histologically marked by infiltration of the nevus by lymphocytes or fat cells or by differentiation into neural structures.

A few variants of the benign nevus deserve mention. The Spitz nevus was originally called benign juvenile melanoma. It occurs in children and young adults usually on the head, neck or upper extremities as a small, solitary, dome-shaped dermal nodule, which is often red in colour. The lesion can be histologically alarming to the novice pathologist but the histological features are well recognized. Clinically and biologically, a Spitz nevus is just another acquired nevus.

The pigmented spindle cell nevus is a distinct clinico-pathological entity which occurs as a small, solitary, deeply pigmented well circumscribed lesion on the extremities and trunk usually of young women. The intense pigmentation is sometimes mistaken for a superficial spreading malignant melanoma. Histologically, a junctional or compound nevus composed of spindle cells arranged parallel to the epidermis is seen.

The blue nevus occurs on the dorsal surface of the hands or feet as a small, solitary, slightly raised, dome-shaped lesion. Histologically, it is composed of dense deposition of pigment in dermal melanophages almost obscuring the melanocytes in the background.

The cellular blue nevus occurs as a dome-shaped blue coloured lesion on the back or buttocks. On microscopical examination, a tumour composed of interweaving fascicles of spindle cells is seen. Melanin pigment can be easily missed and is present in only a few cells and the lesion can be mistaken for a leiomyoma or a dermatofibroma.

In its typical form, the congenital nevus is irregular, hair bearing and larger than a benign nevus, occasionally occupying one half of the trunk or an entire extremity. Histologically, compound and dermal patterns are seen. The dermal component is more extensive than in an acquired nevus with extension into the subcutaneous fat. Involvement of the adnexal structures and perineurium is typical but does not imply malignancy.

DYSPLASTIC NEVUS

The concept of dysplastic nevus is a confusing one to many clinicians and pathologists. It arose from the observation that individuals with a strong family history of melanoma may exhibit clinically atypical nevi sometimes in large numbers. Indeed large numbers of melanocytic nevi in any individual increases their risk of developing malignant melanoma. As well as being clinically odd (large, irregular margin, asymmetric pigmentation) it was noticed that these nevi were also atypical histologically and seemed to show features intermediate between common benign nevi and melanoma. This type of nevus is not confined to "melanoma families" however and does occur sporadically. Affected individuals do have an increased melanoma risk. It is therefore an important diagnosis but unfortunately there has been much controversy amongst pathologists regarding diagnostic criteria and the definition of this entity. This argument has even extended to the nomenclature and it has been recommended that the term dysplastic nevus be abandoned in favour of nevus with architectural disorder and/or cytologic atypia.

MALIGNANT MELANOMA

Malignant melanoma is a serious public health problem with a rising incidence in the United Kingdom. The association with sun exposure in fair-skinned individuals is well known.

The radial and vertical growth phase is the single most important concept in the biology and prognosis of malignant melanoma. The radial growth phase is horizontal spread of the malignant cells along epidermis and the dermo-epidermal junction. Nests of dermal cells may infiltrate the papillary dermis and the superficial plexus but are never larger than those at the junction and there are no mitoses. When a melanoma consisting entirely of the radial growth phase is completely excised, the tumour is completely cured. The radial growth phase can progress to the vertical growth phase which is an ominous development as it represents growth of a clone of cells capable of metastasis. Histologically, the vertical growth phase is recognised by the formation of expansile dermal nodules of atypical melanocytes. The nodules are larger than the nests present in the epidermis or the dermo-epidermal junction and mitoses may be present.

Four variants of malignant melanoma are typically described:

- the superficial spreading melanoma
- lentigo maligna melanoma

- nodular melanoma

- acral lentiginous melanoma .

Lentigo maligna occurs in sun-exposed skin of elderly individuals. Superficial spreading melanoma occurs in all age groups and although associated with sun exposure, is not limited to sun-exposed skin (Figure 4.12). The acral lentiginous melanoma occurs on the palmar, plantar, ungual and subungual regions. It accounts for only 10% of melanomas in Caucasians but is the commonest form of melanoma in the African and Japanese population. Although the biological characteristics are not different from the superficial spreading melanoma, the acral lentiginous melanoma is often diagnosed late in its natural history; this may be partly due to the presence of thickening and hyperkeratosis of the overlying epidermis which may mask the true appearances.

The superficial spreading melanoma, lentigo maligna and acral lentiginous melanoma begin as, and consist predominantly of, a radial growth phase. A vertical growth phase may be heralded by the rapid appearance of a dermal nodule on a long standing pigmented papule. Nodular malignant melanoma starts off with a vertical growth phase apparently without a preceding radial growth phase and carries a poor prognosis.

Depth of infiltration is the most important prognostic indicator in malignant melanoma and is determined by using the Breslow measurement for thickness of a melanoma. Tumours less than 0.76 mm rarely metastasise whereas those above 1.5 mm in thickness have a very high risk of metastases.. Tumours between 0.76 mm and 1.5 mm have an intermediate risk of metastasis. It is most important to remember that the diameter of a lesion has no correlation to the Breslow thickness. It is perhaps superfluous to say that any melanoma needs to be adequately excised in its entirety, as surgery is the only effective treatment.

CYTOPATHOLOGY

Organized cervical screening began over 20 years ago in North America and Europe but not all programmes showed the same level of organization and coverage of the target population. In countries such as Iceland, Finland, Sweden and parts of Denmark where the target population had been almost completely covered, there was a demonstrable decrease in both the incidence and mortality of invasive cervical cancer. In Britain, screening has been operating since 1964 but a decrease in incidence and mortality was not demonstrated, largely because the screening programmes were not organised enough to reach the target population or ensure an adequate follow-up. It has been shown that many women presenting with invasive cervical carcinoma have never had a cervical smear.

In November 1987, a report of the Intercollegiate Working Party made recommendations for a nationwide screening programme that would ensure effective and wide coverage of the target population and thorough follow-up. Emphasis was laid on the role of adequate educational, laboratory and administrative facilities for a successful programme that would produce significant results. The total number of women screened in England in 1992/93 was over 1.5 million which represents an increase of 31.4% since 1991/92 and 67.5% since 1989/90.

Cervical screening is now also reaching those women most at risk of developing invasive cancer. This improvement has largely been brought about by the use of a computerised call/recall system by almost all health authorities and the introduction of a GP contract system. Payments to GPs for cervical screening are triggered on reaching 50-80% coverage of the target population. By October 1993, 83% of GPs had reached the 80% target.

RATIONALE FOR SCREENING

Cervical cancer follows breast cancer as the second commonest cancer in women in the world: 77% of all cases occur in developing countries with the highest incidence in China, Latin America and the Carribean.

The UK has the second highest incidence of cervical cancer and one of the highest death rates in the European Economic Community (EEC). In 1988, 5,000 new cases of invasive carcinoma of the cervix were registered in the UK, making it the eighth commonest cancer in women of all ages and the most common cancer in women under 35 years of age. The significance of these statistics is acknowledged by the government in its 'Health of the Nation' policy which aims to reduce invasive cervical cancers by at least 20% by the year 2000 from 150 per million women in 1986 to no more than 120 per million women.

In England and Wales, there is a strong North/South gradient, the highest risk being in the Northern counties. The strongest risk factors for cervical cancer are related to sexual behaviour. Early age at first intercourse and multiple sexual partners increase the risk of cervical cancer. The incidence is higher in lower socio-economic groups. There is a definite aetiological role of human papilloma virus (HPV) in cervical cancer. This is best demonstrated by the integration of HPV viral DNA into the human genome as detected by sensitive *in-situ* hybridisation techniques. Many HPV types are known but those consistently associated with cervical cancer are types 16, 18 and 31 which are therefore known as high risk types. HPV infection is not always necessary or sufficient to cause cervical cancer and other factors seem to be involved. Cigarette smoking doubles a woman's risk of developing cervical cancer and it is thought that a chemical in cigarette smoke adversely affects immunity in the cervix vital for protecting against the papilloma virus.

Cancer of the cervix has been strongly linked epidemiologically to sexual behaviour. This does not however imply that sexually inactive women cannot develop cervical cancer and should be exempt from regular screening. Preventive measures which would include a change in social customs and habits would be impossible to implement even if there were health gains. There is, however, strong biological evidence that invasive cancer of the cervix arises from a sequential progression of preinvasive dysplastic changes occurring in the surface epithelium in the transformation zone. This is best illustrated by a well known study from New Zealand where women with severe dysplastic changes who were treated conservatively developed invasive cervical cancer. The cure rate for cervical cancer depends on the stage at presentation and is over 99% for precancerous lesions. The rationale for screening arises from an ability to sample the transformation zone and to diagnose dysplastic changes by cytological examination. The test is sufficiently sensitive for a population screening progamme to justify the costs involved.

ORGANIZATION OF THE NATIONAL SCREENING PROGRAMME

Since 1st April 1988, it has been the responsibility of District Health Authorities (DHAs) to ensure that all women between 24-60 years of age are invited for screening at least once every five years. The Family Health Services Authority (FHSA) maintains lists of the target population; inviting them to have a smear requires complex organization and collaboration between GPs, Family Planning Clinics (FPC) and other agencies involved in primary care. The FHSA maintains a register of the target women based on GP practice lists and usually sends out invitation letters although some practices take on this role. An important part of the process involves the transfer of test results from the laboratory to the FHSA computers to ensure appropriate recall. Recall is particularly challenging in inner city areas due to population mobility and considerable numbers of women who are simply not registered.

Almost all DHAs now operate a computerised call/recall system with most health authorities operating a 3 year recall system. It has been clearly shown in the Nordic studies that the success of a screening programme depends on complete coverage of the target population rather than the frequency of screening. A woman screened regularly at 5 year intervals between 20-64 years would undergo nine smears in her life time with a 83.3% reduction in her risk for developing cervical cancer. Increasing the frequency of screening to 3 years offers an additional 7% protection and increases the number of smears in the woman's lifetime to 15. The frequency of recall therefore has to strike a balance between the protection offered and the cost incurred by the health service and the community.

The National Screening Programme has benefitted enormously from concerted efforts to ensure complete coverage, standardised reporting and fail-safe follow-up procedures. Not all questions have been resolved. It is not certain whether younger women or those at high risk should be screened more frequently. Opportunistic smears from sexually active women under 20 years and from women over 64 years are welcome. Women who have had a total hysterectomy for benign disease do not require screening. Women with a hysterectomy and preservation of the cervix require routine screening.

THE PATHOLOGY OF CERVICAL CANCER AND CERVICAL INTRAEPITHELIAL NEOPLASIA

Cervical intraepithelial neoplasia (CIN) is now a well accepted term to encompass the previously used terms of dysplasia and carcinoma-in-situ. The term is conceptually logical as it recognises the continuity of the disease process from the earliest dysplastic changes to the development of an invasive tumour. It has also eliminated the diagnostic confusion that arose between severe dysplasia and carcinoma-in-situ.

The abnormality seen in cervical biopsy specimens is described as dysplasia to denote the architectural as well as cellular pathology. The abnormality is called dyskaryosis when observed in cytology smears to denote the nuclear changes. Dyskaryotic cells are distinguished from normal squamous epithelial cells by an abnormal nuclear/cytoplasmic ratio, irregular nuclear outline and abnormal chromatin structure. Dyskaryosis is classified as mild, moderate or severe. In mild dyskaryosis, the nuclear abnormalities are seen in cells resembling superficial or intermediate cells. The nucleus is enlarged with abnormal chromatin but occupies less than half of the cytoplasm. Moderate dyskaryosis shows nuclear abnormality in intermediate or parabasal cells and the nucleus shows more severe changes, occupying half to a third of the cell cytoplasm. Severely dyskaryotic cells usually appear as small, single parabasal cells in which the nucleus occupies at least two-thirds, if not the entire cytoplasm.

CIN or dysplasia is characterised by an increase in the nuclear size with a resultant increase in the nuclear-cytoplasmic ratio, coarsening and irregularity of the nuclear membrane and the nuclear chromatin and increase in the number and size of nucleoli. The nuclear abnormality is accompanied by a loss of polarity and a lack of maturation of the epithelium. Abnormal and increased numbers of mitotic figures are seen. These changes increase in severity with increasing grade of dysplasia. The nuclear changes involve the full thickness of the epithelium irrespective of the grade of the lesion. Therefore abnormal cells can be scraped from the surface. What distinguishes CIN 1 from CIN 2 and CIN 3 is the relative proportion of the epithelium composed of undifferentiated basal-type cells. When these cells occupy the lower third of the cervical epithelium, the abnormality is classified as CIN 1, when they extend up to two-thirds of the thickness it is called CIN 2. CIN 3 involves the full thickness of the epithelium.

While the continuity of the disease process from CIN 1 to invasive carcinoma is well accepted, it is uncertain whether CIN 1 will invariably progress to CIN 2 and then to CIN 3, and if such a progression is invariable what is the time scale involved? The evidence suggests that at least some cases of CIN 1 and CIN 2 regress. Studies involving follow-up of women with mild dyskaryosis on smears showed that over half of them may revert to normal in a few years, whereas about a fifth persist as mild dyskaryosis and a sixth progress to CIN 3. In one such study, two patients lost to follow-up developed invasive carcinoma. It is estimated that at least 30-40% of cases of CIN 3 will eventually progress to invasive carcinoma if followed up for 20 years. The risk in an individual woman who has CIN 3 or severe dysplasia however, is serious enough to warrant therapy. Furthermore, the severity of changes is not uniform and it is possible that foci of CIN 3 may co-exist with lower grades of abnormality — this forbids complacency with even the lowest grade of nuclear abnormality.

Human papilloma virus (HPV) infection is diagnosed on a smear by the presence of cells with nuclear abnormalities containing a large, well-defined perinuclear vacuole or halo.

This cell is called a koilocyte. The koilocytic nucleus is enlarged and hyperchromatic with an irregular nuclear membrane and clumped chromatin; binucleation is a common feature. These changes can resemble those of dyskaryosis and have to be interpreted with caution in the presence of HPV infection. Koilocytes are also seen on biopsy specimens and are associated with an abnormal maturation of the epithelium. Dyskaryosis and koilocytosis often coexist.

TECHNIQUE FOR TAKING A CERVICAL SMEAR

The technique of taking a smear is well described in a video prepared by the British Society for Cervical Cytology (BSCC) entitled, 'Taking cervical smears'. The aim is to scrape off the surface epithelium from the entire circumference of the transformation zone, as dysplastic changes are first observed there. Good visualisation of the cervix is essential and therefore a speculum of suitable size should be used. No one type of spatula is ideal for all women. The Aylesbury spatula which has an expanded tip provides good quality smears. In patulous or multiparous women a broader spatula may be better.

The cytobrush can be used to obtain a sample after a smear has been prepared from scrapings of the spatula (N.B. put both specimens on one slide as failure to do so could double our workload at a stroke!). The cytobrush causes more bleeding and provides scanty smears and is not the method of choice for primary screening. It is useful when the cervix has been distorted by previous surgery, in some postmenopausal women with a tight os and in women who have consistently had inadequate smears. The spatula or brush should be completely rotated through 360 degrees to sample the entire transformation zone. Contrary to popular belief, wiping off excess exudate or mucus from the surface of the cervix does not affect the quality of the smear. In the screening context manual vaginal examination should not be performed prior to smear-taking as lubricant or blood will obscure the cytological features.

From the laboratory point of view, the smear should be adequate, well spread and properly fixed, correctly labelled and accompanied by a properly filled out request form (HMR 101/5). Glass slides with frosted ends allow proper labelling which should be done in pencil as pen and ball point inks dissolve in the fixative. The patient's name and date of birth should be entered on the frosted end of the slide on the same side as the smear. The recommended fixative is ethanol (90%). Slides can be transported in a pot containing the same fixative which should cover the entire slide. Commercially available spray fixatives, e.g., carbowax, are in wide use as they are more convenient and provide satisfactory fixation. Air-drying and improper fixation produce artefacts in nuclear morphology and thus cause difficulty in interpretation.

SCREENING OF SMEARS

A District General Hospital (DGH) serving a population of 250,000 may expect to receive at least 25,000 cervical smears to cover a 5 year call/recall programme. The Royal College of Pathologists recommends that a DGH laboratory handling 25,000 slides per annum should be staffed by the equivalent of 1.5 whole-time cytopathologists.

The smear is stained by the Papanicolaou method and is screened by a cytoscreener who decides whether there is any abnormality in the smear. Abnormal smears are then checked and signed out either by a senior Medical Laboratory Scientific Officer (MLSO)/Biomedical scientist or more usually a pathologist. An average cervical smear contains between 50,000 and 300,000 cells and it takes on average 5 minutes to screen a single slide. It is recommended that no more than 12 smears should be screened in one hour. Screening of smears is done either by an MLSO or a cytoscreener. To be eligible, the MLSO is required to have one year's training along with a degree in biomedical sciences or two years training without a degree. A cytoscreener has to obtain a certificate of competence from the British Society for Clinical Cytology (BSCC).

An adequate smear is one that has sampled the whole circumference of the transformation zone. Inclusion of the transformation zone is confirmed by the presence of endocervical or metaplastic cells with or without mucus. However, it is the responsibility of the person taking the smear to ensure adequacy or complete sampling as it is not possible to ascertain, even in the presence of endocervical cells, whether the entire circumference or only part of the transformation zone has been sampled. The BSCC has laid down guidelines to determine adequacy of a smear but it is difficult to adhere to these in some circumstances. There are no reliable indicators of transformation zone sampling in post-menopausal women and those who have had a cone biopsy where it may be more appropriate to ascertain adequacy by acceptable cellularity.

DIAGNOSTIC CATEGORIES AND FOLLOW-UP SCHEDULE

The smear results are reported as categories 1 - 6 in Section 22 of the HMR 101/5 form. Any specific infection detected on the smear is reported in Section 23. Section 24 is used to suggest management. An inadequate smear or diagnostic category 1 can result from inadequate sampling, too thick or too thin a smear that obscures cellular detail, drying of smear before fixation or improper fixation. Cellular detail may be obscured by a heavy inflammatory exudate containing many neutrophils or too much blood resulting in a diagnosis of an 'inadequate' smear. Colposcopy may be indicated after 2 - 3 consecutive inadequate smears.

A negative smear does not show any nuclear abnormality and routine recall after three years is recommended. A patient with the first borderline or mild dyskaryosis report is followed up with a smear after six months. Two consecutive borderline or mild dyskaryosis smears are usually referred for colposcopy. Patients with moderate or severe dyskaryosis are referred for colposcopy. Following treatment for CIN, patients with negative smears have to be followed up annually for five years before returning to a routine three-year recall.

It is very important to be aware that the interpretation of smears is subjective and suffers from inter-observer variation. Smears can be especially difficult to interpret at the lower end of the spectrum of CIN. It is sometimes very difficult to distinguish between HPV infection associated with CIN 1 and HPV infection occurring alone. HPV infection by itself i.e. not associated with CIN 1/borderline is not an indication for more frequent screening. When HPV infection is associated with CIN, the woman should be managed according to the grade of the CIN. In practice, it is rare for HPV infection to occur without changes of CIN. The term borderline may be used when nuclear changes cannot be ascribed to HPV alone but fall short of CIN 1. The criteria for diagnosis of HPV infection should be strictly adhered to because of the social implications of a wrong diagnosis. The term borderline is also used when it is impossible to decide whether nuclear changes represent early CIN or are merely reactive in nature. This term more accurately describes the diagnostic dilemma than the previously used label of 'inflammatory smear ' a term which should no longer be used in the reporting of cervical smears.

There is usually good correlation between severe dyskaryosis and the finding of CIN 3 on a biopsy but the diagnostic accuracy is less at the lower end of the spectrum. There is generally poor correlation between a single cervical smear showing mild dyskaryosis and biopsy results. Similarly, inter-observer agreement is high for severe dyskaryosis but not so for mild and moderate dyskaryosis. In one study, follow-up smears of patients with mild dyskaryosis showed that 33% were negative, 23% were borderline and 44% showed dyskaryosis, one third of these being of a higher grade. Follow-up of smears of those diagnosed as having borderline changes showed that 75% of these were subsequently negative, 18% showed persistent borderline changes and only 7% were dyskaryotic.

In another series, 29% of smears reported as borderline dyskaryosis and 41% of those with mild dyskaryosis showed CIN 2 or CIN 3 on biopsy. This underscores the importance of follow-up of the lower grades of dyskaryosis because they frequently co-exist with higher grades. In this context, a single negative diagnosis is a non-diagnosis; two consecutive negative smears are more accurate predictors of the absence of the dyskaryosis. The extent of the cervical epithelial lesion is an important determinant in the correlation between cytological findings and histological diagnosis. In general, the more extensive the lesion, the greater the chance of finding a more severe abnormality.

Candidiasis, trichomonal and herpes simplex infections can be diagnosed on a cervical smear. Candida appears as thin pink non-branching strands corresponding to fungal pseudohyphae associated with spores. Candidiasis is commoner in pregnancy and in women taking oral contraceptives. The infection causes vulvovaginitis with intense itching and a thick white discharge. *Trichomonas vaginalis* is a protozoon which is usually but not invariably sexually transmitted. It causes an acute vaginitis and cervicitis and is associated with a thin, watery discharge. The pathogen appears as an ovoid greyish-blue structure containing an oval nucleus. The nucleus may not always be easy to see and the parasite may then be mistaken for karyolytic debris. The smear from an affected case is usually teeming with neutrophils and a vigorous search for trichomonas should be made in such a case.

Herpes simplex infection is usually caused by the sexually transmitted type 2 virus, Herpes genitalis. It is diagnosed by the presence of multinucleated cells with enlarged nuclei that have a ground-glass appearance due to the presence of virions. The chromatin is pushed to the periphery of the nucleus against the nuclear membrane.

FURTHER READING

SKIN BIOPSIES

Slater D. Performance of skin biopsies by general practitioners BMJ 1991; 303:1472

Godfrey E, Watkiss M, Schnieden H. Health Trends 1990; 2: 57-9.

CERVICAL CYTOLOGY

Walker EM, Hove MJ, Cooper PA. Retrospective review of cervical cytology in females developing massive squamous cell carcinoma. Br J Obstet Gynecol 1983; 90: 1087-91.

Giles JA, Hudson E, Crow J, Williams D, Walker P. Colposcopic assessment of the accuracy of cervical cytology screening. BMJ 1988; 269: 1099-1102.

Laara E, Day NE. Trends in mortality from cervical cancer in the Nordic countries; association with organized screening programmes. Lancet 1987; i: 1247-9.

Walker EM, Dodgson J, Duncan ID. Does mild atypia on a cervical smear warrant further investigation? Lancet 1986; i: 672-3.

Chung AR. Carcinoma-in-situ of the cervix and its malignant potential. A lesson from New Zealand. Cytopathology 1990; 1: 321-328.

Sigurdsson K. Effect of organized screening on the risk of cervical cancer. Evaluation of screening activity in Iceland, 1964-1991. Int J Cancer 1993; 54: 563-70.

Hakama M, Louhivuori K. A screening programme for cervical cancer that worked. Cancer Surveys 1988; 7: 403-16.

Taking Cervical Smears Video and Booklet . British Society for Clinical Cytology, London, 1989.

Report of the intercollegiate working party on cervical cytology screening Royal College of Obstetrics and gynaecology, London, 1987.

McPherson I, Cervical Screening: A Practical Guide. 2nd edition Oxford: Oxford University Press, 1992.

Cancer Research Campaign Factsheets 1994. Cervical Cancer Factsheet 12, Cervical Cancer Screening Factsheet 13, London, 1994.

Wilkinson C, Jones JM, McBride B. Anxiety caused by abnormal result of cervical smear test: a controlled trial. BMJ 1990; 300: 440.

Chapter 5

Haematology

Kate Ryan & Sally Davies

INTRODUCTION

Haematological investigations are frequently requested by primary care practitioners both for the investigation of clinical symptoms and signs and for health screening and promotion. This chapter outlines the laboratory processes by which results are obtained and provides guidance on their interpretation and further patient management.

COLLECTION AND HANDLING OF SPECIMENS

SAMPLE TYPE

Venous blood is preferred for most haematological investigations. Blood taken by skin puncture or capillary methods is sometimes useful for paediatric samples or cases of poor venous access, but may produce less reliable results.

SPECIMEN BOTTLES

Bottles should be filled to the marked line. Incomplete filling or overfilling of bottles can cause significant differences in results, particularly for coagulation investigations, due to dilution of the sample. Most laboratories can provide smaller containers for paediatric use. Unreliable results may be obtained from poorly mixed, incompletely coagulated or haemolysed samples.

Figure 5.1 illustrates a range of specimen bottles and Figure 5.2 indicates the effect of a delay in transit on haematology results.

REFERENCE RANGES

Some examples of the effect of age and sex on the reference range for a number of haematological variables are given in Figure 5.3. It should be noted that the normal adult ratio of neutrophils to lymphocytes is reversed in children until the age of 5-7 years. Ethnic origin should also be taken into account since neutropenia is commonly encountered in healthy subjects of Afro-Caribbean or Indian origin. In order to help laboratories to provide an appropriate reference range, it is essential that patients' clinical and demographic features are supplied on the request forms.

Type	Suitable for:
EDTA	Full blood counts
	Haemoglobin electrophoresis
	Sickle tests
	Red cell folate
	Film examination (including malaria)
Citrate 1:9	Coagulation investigation
Citrate 1:4	ESR
Serum (clotted)	Serum vitamin B_{12} & serum folate

Figure 5.1   Specimen bottles

Storage change	Effect
Red blood cell swelling	Increase in MCV
	Crenation & sphering
	Fall in ESR (reduced rouleaux formation)
White cells - vacuolation & loss of normal nuclear appearance	Loss of accuracy of differential counts
Platelet swelling & disintegration	Falsely high platelet count

Figure 5.2   Effects of delay in transit of sample

- Blood should be transported to the laboratory as soon as possible. Red cell, total leucocyte and platelet numbers are stable for at least 24 hours in EDTA and measurements of haemoglobin concentration are reliable for several days.

THE FULL BLOOD COUNT

Most laboratories rely on automated counters to provide information on cell counts, red cell indices and white cell differentials.

RED CELL INDICES

Haemoglobin (Hb) concentration, red cell count (RCC) and mean corpuscular volume (MCV) are directly measured parameters whilst the packed cell volume (PCV), mean

Reference Ranges for Haematological Values in Children and Adults

Age	Hb (g/dL)	PCV (fL)	MCV (pg)	MCH (g/dL)	MCHC (x10⁹/L)	Average reticulo-cytes (%)	Total WBC range (x10⁹/L)	Absolute neutrophil count (x10⁹/L)	Absolute lymphocyte count (x10⁹/L)	Absolute monocyte count (x10⁹/L)	Absolute eosinophil count (x10⁹/L)
Newborn:											
Full Term	18.4±2.2	0.60±0.07	108±9	35±4	36±2	3.2	9-30	4.5-13.2	2.7-11.0	0.4-3.1	0.2-0.9
1 Year	11.8±0.5	0.39±0.02	78±8	27±4	32±3	0.9	6-15	1.5-7.0	5.0-10.0	0.2-1.5	<0.7
3-6 Years	12.7±1.0	0.37±0.03	87±8	27±3	33±2	1.0	5-21	2.0-6.0	5.5-8.0	0.2-1.5	<0.7
Male adult	16.0±2.0	0.47±0.05	85±8	29.5±2.5	33±2	1.0	4.3-10	2.0-7.5	1.5-4.0	0.2-0.95	<0.7
Female adult	14.0±2.0	0.42±0.05	85±8	29.5±2.5	33±2	1.0	4.3-10	2.0-7.5	1.5-4.0	0.2-0.95	<0.7

PCV = packed cell volume

MCH = mean corpuscular haemoglobin

MCHC = mean corpuscular haemoglobin concentration

WBC = white blood cell count

MCV = mean corpuscular volume

Figure 5.3 Reference ranges for haematological values

corpuscular haemoglobin (MCH) and mean corpuscular haemoglobin concentration (MCHC) are derived, that is calculated values. The MCV is a mean value and a normal result may be obtained in the presence of marked variation in red cell size (anisocytosis); the red cell distribution width (RDW) is an additional parameter that is derived from the size distribution of the red cells and is, therefore, an indicator of anisocytosis. This value may be of use in the differential diagnosis of microcytic anaemias (see below). Derived values are dependent on the direct measurements as follows:

$$PCV = RCC \times MCV$$

$$MCH = \frac{Hb}{RCC}$$

$$MCHC = \frac{Hb}{PCV.}$$

Figure 5.4   Calculation of derived values

The derived values of MCH and MCHC have less clinical importance apart from providing some discriminatory function in the differentiation of iron deficiency and thalassaemia trait (see below). They are, however, useful for laboratory quality control purposes.

WHITE CELL COUNTS

Automated counters recognise leucocytes as nucleated cells. Differentials are obtained on the basis of relative nuclear size to the cell, nuclear complexity, and the presence of cytoplasmic granules.

FACTITIOUS RESULTS

- Factitious results may be due to certain characteristics of the blood sample.

- Some of these may be recognised by a deviation from the pattern of   related parameters or in relation to other investigations. Blood film examination is particularly important in this context.

- Factitious results should be recognised by the laboratory and the results adjusted accordingly.

Some examples of factitious results are shown in Figure 5.5

- **Falsely high haemoglobin results:** this may be seen with increased turbidity of the sample such as occurs with hyperlipidaemias or very high leucocyte counts. Both also result in high values for MCH and MCHC.

- **Red cell counts:** red cell counts may be increased in the presence of extreme leucocytosis or may be falsely low in cases of gross microcytosis or red cell fragmentation. In addition to a low count, red cell agglutination will result in a falsely high MCV and MCH.

- **Differential white cell counts:** storage changes may affect the differential white cell count so that neutrophils can be misread as monocytes. In most cases the instrument will flag abnormalities which ensures that a blood film is examined within the laboratory.

- **Platelet counts:** artificially elevated platelet counts may arise when particles of a similar size, such as red cell fragments, are present. Faulty low platelet counts are most often the result of partially clotted samples or undetected fibrin clots, but may be due to the presence of platelet aggregates. Occasionally large platelets may be excluded from the count. Film examination will generally determine the validity of the count.

Figure 5.5   Examples of factitious results

FILM EXAMINATION

Each laboratory will have defined criteria for the examination of a blood film. These vary between laboratories depending on the clinical workload and the accuracy of their automated counter.

Such criteria include:

- clinically significant deviation of measured parameters from reference ranges

- certain patient groups e.g., haematological or neonatal patients

- clinical history suggestive of haemolytic or haemoglobin disorders, since the instruments are unable to pick up certain morphological abnormalities e.g., red cell inclusions and abnormalities of shape

- examination for instances where abnormalities have been 'flagged' by the counter.

Figure 5.6   Criteria for the examination of a blood film

The accuracy of counters has allowed a significant reduction in the number of manual white cell differentials performed such that an average District General Hospital will examine films from approximately 20-30 % samples, although teaching hospitals with specialised units may examine many more. Film comments are added by the laboratory staff. A guide to common morphological comments and their meaning is given in Figure 5.8. Most laboratories, in addition, communicate very abnormal results directly with the requesting doctor.

INTERPRETATION OF RESULTS

ANAEMIA

It is convenient to classify anaemias according to the MCV. This indicates the possible underlying causes and appropriate avenues of further investigation (see Figure 5.9).

MICROCYTIC ANAEMIA

Causes	Comments
Iron deficiency	
Bleeding	MCV, MCHC & MCH reduced
Increased physiological demand e.g., infancy, adolescence & pregnancy	Film: hypochromic, microcytic cells with poikilocytosis (variable shape), elliptocytosis (pencil cells) and anisocytosis (variable size).
Diet e.g., vegetarian	
Chronic disease	Unresponsive to iron therapy
	Refer for investigation as appropriate

Figure 5.7   Causes of microcytic anaemia

- Iron deficiency is the most common cause of microcytic anaemia and is often encountered during investigation for fatigue

- Early iron deficiency may present with normal indices and iron studies may be needed

- If there is a clear cause of iron deficiency e.g., menorrhagia, the measured indices do not need confirmation

- Iron studies are needed if there is doubt about diagnosis or failure to respond to therapy with iron

- Where there is no obvious cause refer for investigation of peptic ulcer, gastrointestinal tumours, malabsorption, etc.

Red cell finding	Significance
Microcytes	Fe deficiency, thalassaemia
Macrocytes	Alcohol, liver disease, B_{12}/folate deficiency
Polychromasia	Reticulocytosis, e.g., haemolysis, bleeding, haematinic therapy
Elliptocytes	Fe deficiency (pencil cells), hereditary elliptocytosis
Sickle cells	Sickle cell disease
Target cells	Fe deficiency, hyposplenism, liver disease, haemoglobinopathies
Spherocytes	Immune haemolysis, hereditary spherocytosis
Poikilocytosis	Abnormal cell shape; various anaemias
Tear drop cells	Myelofibrosis, myeloprofilerative diseases
Schistocytes or red cell fragments	Microangiopathic haemolytic anaemia, e.g., DIC, carcinoma, thrombotic thrombocytopenic purpura
Blister cells	Oxidative haemolysis, e.g., in G6PD deficiency
Crenated cells	Artefact, age-related, EDTA effect
Howell-Jolly cells	Hyposplenism e.g., coeliac disease, post splenectomy
Agglutination	Presence of agglutinins, e.g., mycoplasma infection
Rouleux	Viral infections, increased plasma proteins - multiple causes (see text under ESR)
Dimorphic picture	Haematinic therapy, sideroblastic anaemia
Nucleated red cells	Severe anaemia (except aplastic), myelofibrosis, carcinomatosis, haemolytic disease of newborn

White cell finding	Significance
Reactive lymphoctes	Viral infection
Atypical lymphocytes	Infectious mononucleosis, viral infections, toxoplasmosis
Plasma-Turk cells	Severe bacterial, viral, or protozoal infections, myeloma
R Shift	Hypersegmented neutrophils, e.g., megaloblastic anaemia
L Shift	Immature myeloid cells; severe pyogenic infections, leukaemoid reactions, CML and myeloproliferative disorders
Smear cells	Chronic lymphocytic leukaemia
Toxic granulation	Infections and inflammatory processes
Leucoerythroblastic	Immature red & white cell precursors; myelofibrosis, malignant marrow infiltration
Pelger Huet anomaly	Hereditary, myeloid leukaemia, myelodysplasia

Figure 5.8   Common blood film abnormalities and their significance

Investigation and Management of Anaemia

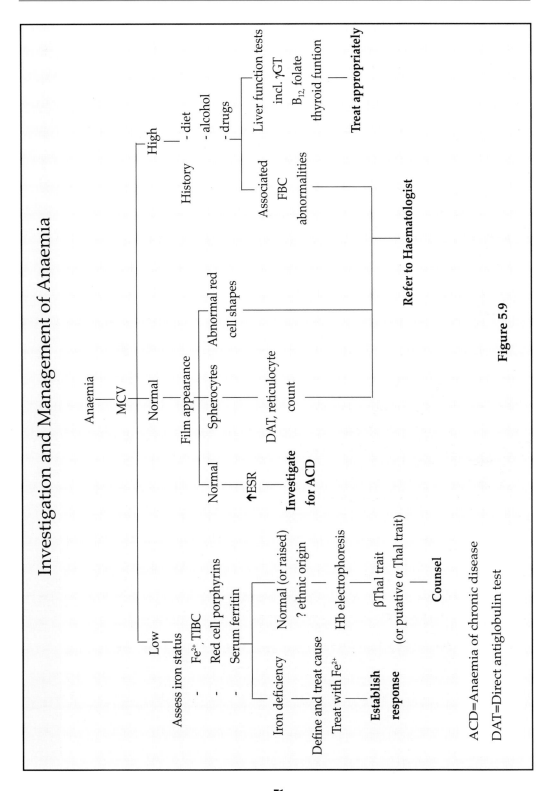

Figure 5.9

ACD=Anaemia of chronic disease

DAT=Direct antiglobulin test

TREATMENT

Oral iron usually increases haemoglobin by 1 g/dL every ten days.

Failure may be due to:

- non-compliance

- ongoing bleeding

- malabsorption

- anaemia of chronic disease

Patients should be re-evaluated clinically and referred for investigation as appropriate.

Persistence of microcytosis following iron treatment may also indicate an underlying *thalassaemia trait*. This should be considered in patients of the appropriate ethnic origin, especially Mediterranean, if they have a persistently low MCV and MCH in the presence of a normal or near normal Hb and MCHC. A further clue may be a raised RCC and a low RDW. If thalassaemia is suspected, the patient should be referred to the local haematologist for investigation by haemoglobin electrophoresis and zinc protoporphyrin studies. Counselling should be arranged by liaison between the GP and the haematologist.

ASSESSMENT OF IRON STATUS

IRON AND TOTAL IRON BINDING CAPACITY

Iron deficiency is the commonest cause of anaemia and occurs due to the body's limited ability to absorb iron, while loss due to bleeding is frequent. In the early stages of iron deficiency, body stores become depleted with little effect on the red cell indices. In the later stages, iron deficiency is reflected in a reduction in serum iron and an increased iron binding capacity. Iron deficiency ultimately leads to changes in red cell morphology with anaemia. Assessment of iron status is usually performed by measuring serum iron and total iron binding capacity (TIBC) the latter being a measure of transferrin, the protein by which iron is transported in the plasma. A summary of the changes in serum iron and TIBC in the investigation of microcytic anaemias in shown in Figure 5.10.

	Iron Deficiency	Chronic inflammation or malignancy	Thalassemia trait α or β	Sideroblastic anaemia
MCV MCH	Reduced related to severity of anaemia	Low normal or mild reduction	All reduced, very low for degree of anaemia	Very low in congenital type MCV often raised in acquired type
Serum iron	Reduced	Reduced	Normal	Raised
TIBC	Raised	Reduced	Normal	Normal
Serum ferritin	Reduced	Normal or raised	Normal	Raised

Figure 5.10   Investigation of microcytic anaemia

FERRITIN

Iron is normally stored in the body as ferritin, a small fraction of which circulates in blood. The concentration of serum ferritin is directly related to tissue stores and levels vary depending on age and sex. In the latent stages of iron deficiency, serum ferritin is reduced whilst overt iron deficiency is generally associated with very low levels. Unfortunately the serum ferritin is raised in acute and chronic disorders such as liver disease, inflammation or malignancy, which limits its use as a diagnostic test as iron deficiency may be masked in these conditions.

Advice from a haematologist should be sought if the results and clinical picture disagree, as occasionally bone marrow estimation of iron stores and utilisation will be required. Serum ferritin levels are generally more accurate than iron and TIBC for the assessment of iron status. They are, however, more time consuming and expensive to measure.

Some laboratories are now adopting assay of **red cell protoporphyrins** for the diagnosis of iron deficiency. An accumulation of these red cell metabolites develops in iron deficiency due to the failure of incorporation of iron in the final stages in the pathway of haem synthesis. The assay is simple to perform and is performed on EDTA specimens. High levels are seen in iron deficiency while borderline raised levels are seen in *anaemia of chronic disease* (ACD), usually accompanied by a raised serum ferritin. We have found this assay to be accurate and popular among primary care practitioners, providing a rapid diagnosis of iron deficiency and helping to distinguish those patients with thalassaemic traits.

Serum ferritin concentrations are increased in patients with haemochromatosis although in the early stages of iron accumulation, an increased serum iron and reduced TIBC is a more sensitive index of iron overload.

NORMOCYTIC ANAEMIA

The commonest causes of a normocytic normochromic anaemia are chronic disease, infections, inflammatory disorders and neoplastic disorders. This is called the anaemia of chronic disease (ACD).

- A more severe anaemia may be seen in renal failure or if the patient develops iron deficiency or bleeding

- Some patients with long-standing ACD may develop a microcytic picture (without being iron deficient) because of impaired delivery of iron to developing erythroblasts

- Haemolysis may be due to inherited or acquired causes and patients should be referred, taking into account a history of prescribed drugs (Figure 5.12).

Causes	Comments
Anaemia of chronic disease (ACD) e.g., chronic infections, inflammatory disorders, neoplasia	Mild to moderate normochromic, normocytic anaemia Reduced serum iron & TIBC Normal/increased ferritin (iron stores) 'Underproduction' anaemia; reticulocyte count inappropriately low for anaemia ESR may be raised
Acute bleeding	Before changes of iron deficiency have appeared Platelet count often raised Reticulocyte count raised
Haemolysis	Film: spherocytes, red cell fragments, sickle cells Reticulocyte count raised Drugs can cause haemolysis

Figure 5.11   Causes of normocytic anaemia

MACROCYTIC ANAEMIA

This is characterised by an increase in mean red blood corpuscle size (macrocytosis) with an increase in MCV. The following points should be noted:

- An increase in MCV above the reference range should always be investigated

- Initial investigations include serum vitamin B_{12} and folate and liver function tests (including γGT); if these are normal, advice should be sought from a local haematologist

- Vitamin B_{12} or folate deficiency may develop insidiously.

Common clinical features of vitamin B_{12} deficiency include:

- weakness and lethargy

- breathlessness

- tingling in hands and feet

- sore mouth or tongue

- mood disturbance with irritability.

Red Cells	Drugs
Iron deficiency (GI blood loss)	Aspirin, non-steroidal anti-inflammatory agents
Immune haemolysis	α methyl DOPA, penicillin
Oxidative haemolysis (esp. G6PD deficiency)	Dapsone, salazopyrine, primaquine, cotrimoxazole, sulphonamides, ciprofloxacin
White Cells	
Neutropenia / agranulocytosis	Clozapine, antithyroid drugs, sulphonamides, anticonvulsants
Neutrophilia	Corticosteroids
Eosinophilia	Sulphonamides, gold salts
Platelets	
Thrombocytopenia	Thiazides, frusemide, quinine, sulphonamides, gold salts, anti-diabetic drugs, heparin.

Figure 5.12   Effects of drugs on the blood

Causes	Comments
Megaloblastic anaemia due to vitamin B$_{12}$ or folate deficiency	Macrocytosis (MCV raised) may predate symptoms. Neutrophil hypersegmentation ('right shift')
Alcohol abuse	Check γ-glutamyltransferase (γGT)
Liver disease	Acanthocytosis or target cells
Primary haematological disorders e.g., myelodysplasia	Associated abnormal leucocyte & platelet counts

Figure 5.13   Causes of macrocytic anaemia

Less common features of vitamin B_{12} deficiency include:

- neurological features due to subacute combined degeneration of the spinal cord

- dementia

- frank psychiatric manifestations.

TREATMENT

Assessment of the response to specific therapy in megaloblastic anaemia is helpful as further proof of a correct diagnosis and may indicate the underlying pathophysiology. Clinical response is seen within a few days of treatment, while the haematological response, as measured by an increase in reticulocytes, is seen between days 5-6 after the initial dose of treatment. The height of the reticulocyte peak is related to the severity of the anaemia and is followed by a decline in the appearance of hypersegmented neutrophils and a decrease in the MCV. It is important to remember that the MCV will fall rapidly in the most anaemic patients, whilst in mildly anaemic patients, the MCV may take several weeks to return to normal. A failure of response to folate may indicate underlying malabsorption warranting gastrointestinal investigations. Except when there is a very obvious dietary cause for vitamin B_{12} deficiency, patients' ability to absorb vitamin B_{12} should be established (see below).

INVESTIGATION OF MEGALOBLASTIC ANAEMIA

An assessment of vitamin B_{12} and folate status is generally required when symptoms suggest megaloblastic anaemia (see above) or macrocytosis is present. In other situations, low levels of vitamin B_{12} or folate do not necessarily indicate significant clinical deficiency. Samples for assay of vitamin B_{12} or folate should be taken before any specific therapy is given. Microbiological assay methods have now largely been replaced by radioisotope dilution or immunological assays, which are not affected by antimicrobial agents.

LABORATORY ASSESSMENT OF VITAMIN B_{12} STATUS

All patients with clinical vitamin B_{12} deficiency have low cobalamin levels and there is usually a correlation between the serum vitamin B_{12} level and the severity of anaemia. Low vitamin B_{12} levels are found in a high proportion of people whose diet is essentially vegetarian or lacto-vegetarian. The majority of these subjects do not have any evidence of megaloblastic anaemia and are able to absorb vitamin B_{12} normally. A small proportion, however, will go on to develop megaloblastic anaemia over a period of time and vitamin B_{12} supplements should be advised.

Low vitamin B_{12} levels are also found in patients with atrophic gastritis due to impaired vitamin B_{12} absorption although transition to pernicious anaemia is rare. Vitamin B_{12} concentrations fall in pregnancy and about 5% of healthy women will have low vitamin B_{12} concentrations at term which do not require any further investigation. In megaloblastic anaemia of pregnancy, vitamin B_{12} deficiency accounts for about a quarter of patients. Low vitamin B_{12} levels may also be seen in patients with primary folate deficiency and occasionally in iron deficient subjects. Thus, the significance of a low vitamin B_{12} level depends on other accompanying findings. Significant deficiency is likely when other evidence of pernicious anaemia is found, with impaired vitamin B_{12} absorption or in strict lifelong vegetarians.

Dietary deficiency of vitamin B_{12} is relatively rare except in strict vegetarians (vegans). The vast majority of cases of vitamin B_{12} deficiency are due to malabsorption, most frequently due to pernicious anaemia or defective intestinal absorption. An assessment of vitamin B_{12} absorption is made by measurement of urinary excretion of an oral dose of radiolabelled vitamin B_{12}— the Schilling test, or the newer dual isotope method (Dicopac test). In this latter test the relative proportions of the excreted isotopes in the urine enables differentiation of gastric from ileal forms of vitamin B_{12} malabsorption. Apart from convenience, this test has a further advantage in that it is less affected by an incomplete urine collection. The majority of patients with pernicious anaemia will also have evidence of intrinsic factor and parietal cell antibodies.

High serum vitamin B_{12} levels are seen in patients receiving treatment but are of no value in monitoring response to therapy; haemoglobin concentration and reticulocyte count should be used for this purpose. Elevated levels of vitamin B_{12} are also seen in liver disease and in the myeloproliferative disorders.

LABORATORY ASSESSMENT OF FOLATE STATUS
Folate status can be measured by estimation of serum folate and red cell folate. Serum folate is low in folate deficiency but low concentrations are also commonly encountered in ill patients, reflecting reduced dietary intake. Thus, this test is of limited diagnostic value.

A low red cell folate level, however, is unequivocal evidence of folate deficiency and is the consequence of several months of reduced folate supply. Clinically significant folate deficiency is often a combination of a reduced dietary intake together with additional factors such as alcoholism, pregnancy, chronic haemolysis or medication with anticonvulsant drugs. A clinical history and examination is essential in the evaluation of clinical folate deficiency. Where indicated, the patients should be referred for investigation of malabsorption. It should be remembered that increased folate levels with vitamin B_{12} deficiency may indicate a blind loop syndrome. Normal or increased serum folate levels with reduced red cell folate levels are also seen in pernicious anaemia.

POLYCYTHAEMIA

This is characterised by an increase in PCV and may be due to an increase in red cell mass (absolute polycythaemia) or to a decrease in plasma volume (apparent polycythaemia).

Causes	Comments
Absolute polycythaemia	PCV usually >60%
Primary myeloproliferative disorder	Features include: splenomegaly
	raised platelet count
	raised WCC >12.0 x 10^9/L
	raised serum vitamin B$_{12}$
Secondary:	
hypoxic lung disease	Need to be excluded.
renal tumours	
cyanotic heart disease	
Apparent polycythaemia	
Common in obese males	At risk of occlusive vascular
Associated with:	episodes. Treat cause.
diuretic therapy	
alcohol	
hypertension	
stress	
smoking	

Figure 5.14   Causes of polycythaemia

WHITE CELL ABNORMALITIES

Modern automated counters generally give accurate differentials of white cells and serious abnormalities due to leukaemia or other haematological disorders should be flagged by the instrument and confirmed by morphological examination of the blood film. These conditions require specialist investigation which is beyond the scope of the book.

LEUCOCYTOSIS

Leucocytosis is present when the leucocyte count is raised, usually above 10 or 11 x 10^9/L. The increased count is often due to a predominance of one type of white cell, most often neutrophils, with modest increases in members of other series.

Causes	Comments
Neutrophilia Bacterial & other infections	In severe pyogenic infections, immature neutrophils may be seen ('left shift')
Inflammation	Toxic granulation may be present
Chronic myeloid leukaemia & other myeloproliferative disorders	Very high neutrophil count including myelocytes Eosinophil, basophil and platelet counts may be raised
Eosinophilia Allergic & dermatological conditions Drugs (see Figure 5.12) Parasitic infections Hodgkin's disease Vasculitis	Stool examination indicated if no apparent cause of eosinophilia especially in children
Monocytosis Chronic bacterial infections e.g., tuberculosis	Relative monocytosis
Myelomonocytic leukaemia or myelodysplastic syndrome	Absolute monocytosis Splenomegaly & other blood count abnormalities
Lymphocytosis Viral infections (particularly children) Infectious mononucleosis	Atypical lymphocytes - may resemble lymphoblasts Request Monospot or equivalent test
Chronic infections Chronic lymphocytic leukaemia	Relative lymphocytosis Absolute lymphocytosis Lymphocytes >5 x 10^9/L Film: smear cells

Figure 5.15   Causes of leucocytosis

- See Figure 5.3 for reference ranges

- If infection is not apparent in neutrophilia, or persists after treatment, refer for bone marrow examination

- Eosinophilia requires careful history and referral if persistent or no obvious cause.

Many patients with chronic lymphocytic leukaemia are asymptomatic and do not require treatment. Many haematology departments do not confirm the diagnosis until the lymphocyte count is in excess of $10 \times 10^9/L$ or the patient develops lymphadenopathy, splenomegaly or associated cytopenias.

The term **leucoerythroblastic leukaemia** describes a form of anaemia in which nucleated red cells and myeloid precursors appear in the peripheral blood. This finding is seen when the bone marrow is infiltrated by malignant disease, myeloma or myelofibrosis and occasionally in some patients with severe infections. Patients should be referred for clinical evaluation and bone marrow biopsy.

LEUCOPENIA

Causes	Comments
Acute viral infections	Neutropenia and lymphocytopenia. Duration variable & repeat count in convalescent period - usually after 2 to 3 weeks
HIV infection	Persistent neutropenia
Ethnic variation	
Drugs (Figure 5.12)	Take history

Figure 5.16   Causes of leucopenia

- Patients with neutrophil counts below $1.0 \times 10^9/L$ are prone to infection.

- Unexplained neutropenia, particularly if persistent or associated with infections or other haematological abnormalities, should initiate referral to a haematologist for further investigation.

PLATELET ABNORMALITIES

THROMBOCYTOSIS

Causes	Comments
Thrombocytosis Primary e.g., myeloproliferative disorders	Diagnosis likely if splenomegaly or neurological symptoms Primary cause more likely if count >1000 x 10^9/L
Secondary (more common): Infectious or inflammatory disorders	Usually associated with neutrophilia
Bleeding	Usually iron deficient
Hyposplenism/splenectomy	Associated with target cells or Howell Jolly bodies.

Figure 5.17   Causes of thrombocytosis

The distinction between a primary and secondary thrombocytosis is quite difficult in clinical practice and borderline raised counts, in the absence of underlying disease, symptoms or associated haematological abnormalities, should be monitored at regular intervals and referred for further investigation if the platelet count is in excess of 600 x 10^9/L.

THROMBOCYTOPENIA
Thrombocytopenia may arise due to a defect of platelet production or reduction in platelet survival or a combination of these two. Disorders of platelet production due to bone marrow aplasia or malignant infiltration will usually be associated with other haematological abnormalities.

Causes	Comments
Viral infections	Usually resolves within a few weeks
Drugs e.g., NSAIDs, diuretics, alcohol excess	Likely drugs should be stopped
Liver disease	Perform liver function tests (LFTs)
Immune thrombocytopenia (often following viral infection in children)	Most children will not require specific therapy
Gestational	100-150 x 10^9/L not infrequent in last trimester; does not usually have implications for fetus but check with haematologist if in doubt

Figure 5.18   Causes of thrombocytopenia

- Patients with a platelet count below 50x 10^9/L, from whatever cause, are prone to spontaneous haemorrhage and should be referred for urgent investigation, particularly if bleeding symptoms are present.

- Persistent unexplained thrombocytopenia should be referred for haematological evaluation.

ERYTHROCYTE SEDIMENTATION RATE

The erythrocyte sedimentation rate (ESR) is related to the degree of red cell aggregation which occurs due to the formation of rouleaux in undisturbed, anticoagulated blood when red cells stack together. In normal plasma, rouleaux formation is minimal and the ESR is low. An alteration of plasma proteins following *tissue damage, and during inflammation* and *chronic pathological processes* will increase the rate of rouleaux formation and is the basis for measurement of the ESR as a non-specific test of inflammation.

Causes	Comments
Acute disease (inflammation, tissue damage) due to an increase in acute phase response proteins	ESR raised after one day and subsides within 4 to 6 days after resolution
Chronic disease - due to an increase in IgG	ESR of help in monitoring If very high, consider temporal arteritis, malignancy, chronic infections, paraproteinaemia e.g., myeloma
Pregnancy	ESR raised due to reduced PCV, raised globulin & fibrinogen
Elderly	ESR raised due to reduced plasma albumin concentration

Figure 5.19   Causes of an increased ESR

- Alterations of red cell shape e.g., sickle cell spherocytosis may reduce their ability to form rouleaux and an increase in ESR may be seen in anaemia and some inflammatory conditions which are associated with hypoalbuminaemia.

- Many apparently normal elderly subjects will, however, have ESRs in excess of this range and references values will vary depending on the type of elderly population e.g. hospital or community. As a *screening* test, therefore, the ESR has limited value in the elderly due to the overlap of values in health and disease and results must be interpreted in light of the clinical background.

Upper reference ranges for the ESR (mm/hr) at various ages are:

Age (years)	Male	Female
17-50	10mm/hr	12mm/hr
> 50	14mm/hr	20mm/hr

Figure 5.20   Upper reference ranges for ESR

A falsely reduced ESR is seen in conditions with an elevated PCV or with abnormalities of cell shape such as is encountered with sickle cell disease or marked spherocytosis. Conversely, a falsely increased reading may be seen with anaemia or certain inflammatory conditions associated with hypoalbuminaemia.

As an alternative to the ESR, some laboratories measure plasma viscosity and in most cases there is a direct correlation between them.

RETICULOCYTE COUNT

Reticulocytes are non-nucleated immature red cells containing precipitable ribosomal RNA. Such cells are present in the circulation for approximately 48 hours, gradually losing their ribosome content as the cell matures. Reticulocytes are generally larger than mature cells and appear polychromatic (blue) on routine blood films.

The reticulocyte count:

- is an index of red cell production by the bone marrow

- increases due to increased red cell turnover, due to bleeding or haemolysis, in the presence of anaemia

- rises in response to successful therapy in haematinic deficiencies

- may be low due to, for example, impaired red cell production in aplastic anaemia or chronic haemolysis e.g., parvovirus infection.

Figure 5.21   Role of the reticulocyte count

PARASITIC INFECTIONS

Malaria should be suspected in patients with fever who have recently visited endemic areas. Laboratory diagnosis is made by demonstrating parasites at various stages of their lifecycle in red cells. Thick films, which are generally prepared by the laboratory, enable many more cells to be examined than a thin film and are therefore useful for screening purposes. However, morphological identification of the species of plasmodium is not usually possible from a thick film so thin films should also be examined. An estimate of the number of infected red cells is of clinical value in *Plasmodium falciparum* infections and is related to the incidence of clinical complications. Morphological identification of the malarial species may be difficult if the patient has been inadequately treated. Further samples should be sent for screening if there is a strong clinical suspicion of malaria and initial films are negative.

A useful indicator in malaria infection is the presence of thrombocytopenia which is inversely related to the degree of parasitaemia. In acute infections, blood taken 8-10 hours after the peak of fever is associated with the appearance of mature trophozoites. In chronic infections, samples may be taken at any time and parasites can even be seen during apyrexial stages of the lifecycle. Some antimalarial agents are associated with haemolysis in glucose 6-phosphate dehydrogenase (G6PD) deficient subjects. This is inherited as a sex linked disorder in som individuals of Asian, Mediterranean or African origin and males of the appropriate ethnic groups should be screened prior to therapy. Advice should be taken from the local haematology or infectious diseases departments. Malarial gametocytes may persist for some days following therapy and do not, therefore, necessarily indicate treatment failure.

THE HAEMOGLOBINOPATHIES

The haemoglobinopathies are a family of inherited abnormalities of haemoglobin production either resulting in a reduction or absent production of normal haemoglobin chains i.e. the thalassaemias, or in the production of variant haemoglobin chains - the most common of which is beta S responsible for the HbS of sickle cell disease (SCD). In the trait/carrier/heterozygous state, a person is healthy, while when two abnormal genes are inherited in the homozygous situation, a clinically significant disease can ensue. All people of non-pure North European origin may be affected, but SCD is most common in people from sub-Saharan regions of Africa and in Afro-Caribbeans whilst the thalassaemias are frequently encountered in people from the Mediterranean, Indian sub-continent and the Orient. Haemoglobin types remain the same throughout life so, once a diagnosis has been made, repeat checking is unnecessary.

Diagnosis is by review of the RBC parameters on automated FBC, Hb electrophoresis and quantitation of Hb bands. All of these tests are generally routinely available from haematology laboratories and the results should be provided along with an interpretation as this is a specialised area.

In *beta thalassaemia trait*, there will be a mild anaemia, low MCV, MCH and MCHC with basophilic stippling in the RBCs on film examination in Mediterranean patients. The confirmatory test is to demonstrate an increased HbA_2 level > 3.5%. Definitive diagnosis of *alpha thalassaemia trait* requires DNA analysis, which is expensive and limited in availability. The full complement of haemoglobin alpha genes is four and progressively more severe abnormalities, which can be assessed by laboratory measurements, are associated with inheritance of increasing numbers of abnormal alpha genes.

With the haemoglobin variants, microcytosis in the absence of iron deficiency is rare. The diagnosis of a haemoglobin variant is made by the Hb pattern on electrophoresis and when a band runs as sickle haemoglobin with a confirmatory sickle test.

There are three important times to screen for the haemoglobinopathies:

- all patients from ethnic minorities should be screened for HbS prior to anaesthesia and surgery

- all women of childbearing age from non North European origin should be screened for haemoglobinopathy. Carriers should be counselled as to the genetic implications and offered testing of their partner, follow up counselling and pre-natal diagnosis as appropriate. This can be arranged and carried out within the primary care context, or through the local haematologists or regional clinical genetics service. Guidance on counselling is available in a recent Standing Medical Advisory Committee report

- neonatal screening will establish those babies with clinically significant disease in order to ensure early entry to 'comprehensive care programmes' e.g., penicillin prophylaxis for SCD.

Figure 5.22   Important times to screen for the haemoglobinopathies

ANTE NATAL SCREENING

Most women's initial contact with the health service, on becoming pregnant, will be with primary care. Increasing numbers of practices are now running booking clinics, 'shared care' ante natal programmes or full ante natal care. It is important, therefore, that their doctors arrange the essential screening tests for these women at the appropriate time. Specialist advice should be sought early particularly in the presence of an atypical alloantibody or a couple 'at risk' of genetic disease.

For haematology, this means:

Pre-conceptual/at initial presentation of pregnancy — genetic screening including a full family history and haemoglobinopathy screen. Carriers should be counselled leading to partner call up and testing. When the partner is affected, counselling and pre-natal diagnosis, if appropriate and acceptable should be arranged as soon as possible.

Ante natal booking clinic — the FBC should be checked and investigated if abnormal. The ABO and Rhesus blood groups should be checked and a serum screen for atypical alloantibodies performed. If atypical alloantibodies e.g., anti-D are present, immediate specialist advice should be sought.

Figure 5.23   Ante natal screening

In Rhesus (D) negative women:

- Repeat the serum screen for atypical alloantibodies at 28-30 weeks and seek specialist advice if one has developed.

- If there is haemorrhage or a miscarriage, and if gestation > 12 weeks arrange a Kleihauer test on the maternal sample, and an injection of the appropriate quantity of anti-D.

- Post partum, arrange a blood group on the baby and if Rhesus D+ perform antiglobulin test, Hb and serum bilirubin estimation. If the baby is Rhesus D+, then a Kleihauer test should be arranged on a maternal sample and appropriate quantities of anti-D administered to the mother within 72 hours after delivery.

COAGULATION

THE PATIENT WITH EASY BRUISING OR BLEEDING

This is a common symptom in primary care and in the majority of cases the patient's coagulation function will be normal. Pointers to an inherited or acquired coagulation defect are the type and severity of bleeding, a lifelong history, a family history of bleeding problems or excessive bleeding after haemostatic challenges such as dental procedures, surgery or childbirth. A drug history is also important. Initial investigations should include a full blood count and a coagulation screen. Thrombocytopenia should be managed as outlined above.

The coagulation screen includes an **activated partial thromboplastin time** (APTT), **prothrombin time** (PT) and assessment of fibrinogen level either by a specific assay or by **thrombin time** (TT). Care should be taken in the collection of specimens as outlined above and tests should be normally performed within a few hours. Partial activation of coagulation may occur due to excessive mixing and will shorten clotting times.

The APTT is a functional measure of the intrinsic pathway of coagulation activation. When the APTT is prolonged, the laboratory should perform mixing studies to determine whether it corrects with the addition of normal plasma. Correction implies a deficiency of one or more of the clotting factors whereas a failure to correct is suggestive of the presence of an inhibitor. Patients with a possible coagulation factor deficiency should be referred for specialist investigations as there are implications, not only for the clinical management of surgery and bleeding episodes, but also to enable genetic counselling. It should be remembered that a normal APTT does not exclude carrier status for haemophilia and it may be normal in cases of mild von Willebrand's disease. Patients with a significant family history should be referred regardless of their coagulation screen. The commonest cause of a failure to correct the APTT is the presence of a lupus anticoagulant. Lupus anticoagulants are not only seen in association with systemic lupus erythematosis, but are also present in a number of other immune disorders, in neoplasia or may be an isolated finding. Lupus anticoagulants are a recognised cause of thrombophilia and recurrent miscarriages. The APTT is also used to monitor heparin therapy (see below).

The PT is a measure of the vitamin K dependent clotting factors II, VII, IX and X. A long PT is seen in liver disease, when it may be associated with a prolonged APTT, hypofibrinogenaemia and thrombocytopenia. In the absence of any other haematological abnormalities and normal liver function tests, a prolonged PT may still reflect liver disease, but it may also indicate vitamin K deficiency secondary to malabsorption. The PT is prolonged by the action of the vitamin K antagonist, e.g., warfarin. This forms the basis for anticoagulant monitoring (see below).

A qualitative or quantitative abnormality of fibrinogen will result in a prolongation of the TT. This is often seen in conjunction with liver disease, but may be hereditary, when a family history can usually be elicited.

BLEEDING TIME
A strongly suggestive history of a bruising or bleeding abnormality despite normal blood count and coagulation screen should merit further investigation by a bleeding time. This is a measure of platelet function and interaction with the vessel endothelium.

Acquired abnormalities of platelet function are commonly due to:

- *drugs,* usually aspirin or non-steroidal anti-inflammatory drugs
- garlic and fish oils will also affect platelet function.

Inherited abnormalities leading to a prolonged bleeding time include:

- von Willebrand's disease
- platelet storage pool disorders
- defects of platelet membrane receptors.

Patients should be advised to omit likely drugs 7-10 days prior to the bleeding time being performed. A prolonged bleeding time warrants further investigation using specialist platelet aggregation studies and coagulation assays which should be performed by the haematology laboratory.

MONITORING ANTICOAGULANT TREATMENT

Monitoring of warfarin and other oral anticoagulant drugs is performed by measurement of the international normalised ratio (INR), which is a prothrombin time ratio (normal/control) which has been corrected for the type of thromboplastin used. This method of expression ensures that INR results are equivalent both over time and between laboratories. Guidelines have been produced by the British Society of Haematology for the therapeutic range of INR for various indications. In most indications, an INR of between 2 and 3 is satisfactory whilst for patients with mechanical prosthetic heart valves, recurrent thromboembolic disease or arterial disease, a higher INR of 3-4.5 is currently recommended. Once a patient has been stabilised on oral anticoagulants, the INR should be monitored every 8-10 weeks. Drug interactions are particularly important with oral anticoagulants and may necessitate additional monitoring; a comprehensive list is available in the British National Formulary.

The APTT is not sensitive to the low levels of heparin dosage that are encountered on patients receiving prophylactic doses e.g., post operatively. Patients on higher dose heparin should be monitored in association with an anticoagulant clinic. Treatment with low molecular weight derivatives of heparin, which are increasingly being used for thromboprophylaxis, cannot be monitored by the APTT and a more specific assay is generally required. However, they generally do not require monitoring in this context.

INVESTIGATION OF THROMBOPHILIA.

Thrombophilia can be defined as the familial or acquired disorders of the haemostatic mechanism which are likely to predispose to thrombosis. Many plasma abnormalities have now been associated with thrombophilia. A normal clotting screen does not exclude thrombophilia and patients need referral for specialist investigation. The following list (Figure 5.24) is a guide to patients in whom investigation for thrombophilia should be considered .

- Venous thromboembolism before the age of 40-45 years.

- Recurrent venous thrombosis or thrombophlebitis.

- Thrombosis in unusual sites e.g., cerebral vein, mesenteric vein.

- Unexplained neonatal thrombosis.

- Skin necrosis particularly if on coumarin/anticoagulants.

- Arterial thrombosis before the age of 30.

- First degree relatives of patients with thrombophilic abnormality.

- Patients with a clear family history of venous thombosis.

- Unexplained prolonged activated partial thromboplastin time.

- Patients with recurrent fetal loss, idiopathic thrombocytopenia or SLE.

Figure 5.24   Investigation of thrombophilia

This list is not comprehensive and each patient will need to be considered on an individual basis. Ideally thrombophilic testing should be performed with the patient off warfarin although in high risk cases, adjustment can be made for the warfarin effect.

FURTHER READING

Hoffbrand A V, Pettit J E. Essential Haematology. 3rd Edition. Oxford: Blackwell Scientific Publications 1993.

Dacie J V, Lewis S M. Practical Haematology. 7th Edition. London: Churchill Livingstone 1991.

Hall R, Malia R G. Medical Laboratory Haematology. Oxford: Butterworths 1984.

British Committee for Standards in Haematology. Standard Haematology Practice. Oxford: Blackwell Scientific Publications 1991.

The Thalassaemia Working Party of the BSH General Haematology Task Force. Guidelines for investigation of alpha, and beta thalassaemia traits. J Clin Path 1994; 47: 289-295.

Report of the Standing Medical Advisory Committee on sickle cell disease, thalassaemia and haemoglobinopathies. London HMSO 1993.

The British Society for Haematology. Guidelines on oral anticoagulation: 2nd edition. J Clin Path 1990; 43: 177-183.

British National Formulary. London: British Medical Association. Published annually.

The British Committee for Standards in Haematology. Guidelines on the investigation and management of thrombophilia. J Clin Path. 1990; 43: 703-709.

Chapter 6

Microbiology

John Philpott-Howard

INTRODUCTION

Microbiological tests differ significantly from those of other pathology specialties. This is because an additional factor must be taken into account: the nature of micro-organisms and the special problems that arise during their detection and culture, especially the additional time taken for growth and identification of delicate organisms, or those in low numbers amongst a normal microbial flora. It is worth noting that although culture is more demanding (and is perceived to be somewhat old-fashioned), it is still the gold standard against which newer techniques such as the detection of antigens, antibodies and nucleic acids are measured. Isolation of organisms also provides important information on antimicrobial resistance and epidemiology of infectious diseases which should assist practitioners in their antibiotic prescribing.

Rapid, cheap and accurate near-patient tests are still poorly developed in microbiology, and the best non-culture tests often have specificities and sensitivities in the order of only 85 to 90% compared with culture, even in the hands of experienced staff. In addition, there are other potential problems with near-patients tests, such as lack of safety and quality control (see Apendix I).

Because of the special problems associated with microbiological tests, the laboratory and practitioner should discuss their requirements in order to anticipate and deal with any problems that may arise. In addition to the requirements described on page 94, practitioners should seek the service commitment from their microbiology laboratory listed in Figure 6.1.

- assurance and evidence of a high-quality service

- acceptable turn-around times, e.g., three days for urines and swabs

- telephoning urgent results e.g., isolation of faecal pathogens such as salmonella, shigella & campylobacter; or isolation of group A streptococci from any site

- information on sampling procedures for specific tests e.g., investigation for chlamydia, electron microscopy, sampling for pertussis

- access to a medical microbiologist for advice on diagnostic and therapeutic problems, and infection control

- consultation about reporting of antibiotic sensitivities, and other information

- costs of tests for fundholding practices; arrangements for block contracts.

Figure 6.1   Service commitment from the microbiology laboratory

The laboratory should be able to provide other types of information, for example through a newsletter or the laboratory handbook (Figure 6.2).

- laboratory hours and contact numbers

- antibiotic resistance rates and related problems in the local community

- availability of certain tests in the community e.g., blood cultures

- information on facilities at the laboratory for taking samples from patients, if available

- location of services sometimes provided by different pathology laboratories, e.g., pregnancy tests, malaria films.

Figure 6.2   Information provided by the laboratory

Although some laboratories are able to send results by fax or a computer modem link, microbiological results, particularly those related to sexually transmitted diseases, may contain sensitive information. For example, even negative HIV results are confidential since the patient may not wish others to know that the test has been performed. Suitable arrangements for computer security and confidentiality must therefore be made.

Practitioners should be committed to obtaining the best and most appropriate sample from their patients, before commencing antibiotics. Attention should be paid to the provision of information which will assist the laboratory, and every endeavour should be made to provide all specimens in a safe manner according to current regulations. All urgent work must be arranged by direct contact with the laboratory staff.

SPECIMENS

SPECIMEN CONTAINERS AND LABELS

Specimen containers must be of a type approved by the laboratory for safe transport of blood and body fluids. A vacuum blood container system may be used for most standard diagnostic blood collections but not for other specimens or blood culture. Nearly all microbiological blood tests use tubes without anticoagulant (an important exception is examination for malarial parasites).

LABELLING OF CONTAINERS & SLIDES

Specimen container labels should be completed using a ball-point pen, including the patient's case number, surname, first name and the date when the sample was taken.

PACKAGING OF SPECIMENS BY THE SENDER

Specimen containers must be robust and leak-proof, and not externally contaminated by the contents.

Specimens collected by pathology van or a similar arrangement:

- all specimens must be placed individually in self-sealing plastic bags with the specimen in the sealable compartment and the accompanying form in the adjacent pocket

- the form must not be placed in the same section as the specimen

- glass slides should be placed in an approved rigid container.

Specimens sent by other means, e.g., taxi, courier, Royal Mail, internal post:

There are stringent guidelines which must be followed:

- the specimen is placed in a plastic bag with the form separate or in the special pouch, as described above

- the bag is placed in a rigid cardboard box surrounded by wadding such as cotton wool or paper towels

- the box is then taped and marked 'Biohazard' (or 'Pathological Specimen, Handle with Care') and labelled with the origin address and laboratory destination address.

PACKAGING AND LABELLING OF HIGH RISK SAMPLES

Samples from patients suspected of having hepatitis B or HIV infection must be securely packaged in sealed plastic bags. The request form and specimen should bear 'Danger of Infection' labels and the nature of the risk should be written on the form. The form must be completely separate from the sample, preferably in an opaque envelope to maintain confidentiality in the case of HIV.

SUMMARY OF PROCEDURE FOR SENDING HIGH-RISK SPECIMENS TO PATHOLOGY DEPARTMENTS OR FOR REQUESTING VENESECTION BY A PHLEBOTOMIST

See Appendix II

OROPHARYNGEAL & UPPER RESPIRATORY TRACT INFECTIONS

ACUTE PHARYNGITIS

The throat swab must be taken with reasonable pressure against the fauces and tonsils or tonsillar bed and placed in a tube of transport medium (e.g., Stuart's) which is packaged with the swab. Indications for throat swabs are shown in Figure 6.3.

- severe sore throat

- tonsillitis/pharyngitis

- acute cervical lymphadenopathy

- oral ulceration (herpetic)

- other oral ulceration (gingivitis, Vincent's angina)

- suspected thrush if the diagnosis is uncertain on clinical examination

- screening for carriage of methicillin-resistant staphylococcus aureus (MRSA, together with nose swab - see also page 116); also screening for *Corynebacterium diphtheriae & Neisseria meningitidis* (only at the direction of a consultant in communicable disease control).

Figure 6.3   Indications for a throat swab in general practice

- Gonococcal pharyngitis is rare and swabs must be taken in the genito-urinary medicine clinic and inoculated directly on to selective media; gonococci and meningococci are not sought in routine throat swabs.

- If severe mouth or gingival ulceration is present, either with or without pharyngitis, an ulcer swab can be stained for Vincent's organisms; this request should be stated on the form.

- A swab broken off into viral transport medium is of value for culture of herpes simplex virus from patients with oropharyngeal ulceration. It would be necessary to contact your virology laboratory to obtain the medium, or they may be willing to swab the patient at the laboratory. A slide preparation for electron microscopy could also be useful (see under Miscellaneous sites of infection, page 111).

VIRAL UPPER RESPIRATORY TRACT INFECTIONS

Investigation of viral upper respiratory infections is infrequently performed owing to the cost and lack of specific treatment available. However, if upper respiratory secretions are aspirated into a container the virology laboratory can perform direct immunofluorescence for a wide range of viruses affecting the upper and lower respiratory tract: respiratory syncytial virus, adenovirus, influenza A & B, parainfluenza 1 & 3. Throat washings are unpleasant for children and should only be used if aspiration fails to produce adequate secretions. If a patient presents with significant conjunctivitis and pharyngitis they should be investigated for adenovirus infection by taking a sample of upper respiratory secretions.

Infectious mononucleosis is common in young adults with sore throat and malaise and blood should be sent for the appropriate tests (see Miscellaneous infections, page 111).

Oral **candidosis** can present as a sore throat and mouth, and can be investigated by asking the patient to perform an oral rinse with 10 mL of normal saline, which is then placed into a universal container. A direct swab of the suspected candida lesion is also sent. This is particularly important if the patient has received treatment and relapsed. Respiratory **mycoplasmas** probably do cause a small proportion of infections during epidemic years (every four years) but they are very difficult to culture. Examination of serum for mycoplasma IgM (an ELISA or latex agglutination) can be useful but should be reserved for the investigation of lower respiratory tract infections.

A peritonsillar abscess is normally managed with antibiotics alone without drainage but in any event the patient requires the urgent attention of an ENT surgeon.

Rare causes of pharyngitis include diphtheria, syphilis and leprosy. Any clinical suspicion of diphtheria requires immediate referral to hospital for assessment; do not wait for the results of cultures. Similarly, stridor or other symptoms indicating epiglottitis and other severe infections must be referred immediately to the local hospital.

Laryngeal spasm and obstruction may occur during an attempt to take a throat swab or other sample in such cases.

Throat swabs are not suitable for culture of *Bordetella pertussis;* a pernasal sample should be taken with a flexible wire swab and sent to the laboratory in charcoal transport medium. Telephone the laboratory to inform them (a special culture plate must be prepared).

INTERPRETATION OF CULTURES

A Gram stain is not performed on throat swabs since it is not useful, except for the detection of Vincent's organisms (spirochaetes, *Borrelia vincentii*) in ulcerative pharyngitis. Group A streptococci should be treated when cultured but about 5% of young children are carriers and so the organism may not necessarily be the cause of sore throat. The management of suspected streptococcal sore throat is a problem, and undoubtedly many unnecessary prescriptions are given because viral and streptococcal infections are often clinically indistinguishable. At the present time, streptococcal antigen detection tests are insensitive and so a negative result may still be culture-positive. Group A streptococci are still universally sensitive to penicillin, and are usually sensitive to erythromycin.

Group C & G beta-haemolytic streptococci can cause pharyngitis but some individuals are carriers. As there are no sequelae like those of group A streptococcal infection, if the patient has recovered without treatment there is no reason to attempt to eradicate carriage with antibiotics. *Staphylococcus aureus*, pneumococci or haemophili in a throat swab nearly always represent carriage.

Throat carriage of meningococcus (*Neisseria meningitidis*) may be detected although it is not part of routine culture nor is it necessary to screen close contacts of a case of meningococcal disease (other than in a major outbreak, at the direction of the Consultant in Communicable Disease Control, the CCDC). However, if the organism is cultured from the throat, for any reason, an attempt should be made to eradicate carriage (e.g., with rifampicin).

Anaerobic bacteria are not reported by the laboratory as they are part of the normal flora. A rare septicaemic infection, preceded by sore throat (Lemiérre's disease) is caused by *Fusobacterium necrophorum* but cultures would have to be specially requested.

Some laboratories examine throat swabs routinely for *Corynebacterium diphtheriae* and occasionally the medical microbiologist will contact the GP about suspected colonies of diphtheria bacilli growing on the agar plates. These often turn out to be commensal 'diphtheroids', i.e., other species of corynebacteria, but until the full identity of the organisms is determined it is necessary to confirm that the individual is generally well, and has no clinical evidence of diphtheria.

Herpes simplex virus may be cultured from the oropharynx of an individual recovering from clinical infection. As treatment does not eradicate carriage, isolation of the virus from a patient who has already recovered does not require therapy.

Figure 6.4 summarises the options for the empirical therapy of acute pharyngitis.

Presentation & associated symptoms	Likely causative organism	Management
Acute pharyngitis alone	Viral (rhinovirus, coronavirus etc.) or *Streptococcus pyogenes*	Symptomatic; throat swabs for streptococcal culture
Acute pharyngitis with lymphadenopathy & systemic upset	*Streptococcus pyogenes*	Oral penicillin or erythromycin or cephalosporin
	Epstein-Barr virus or cytomegalovirus	Investigation for glandular fever: Monospot, specific IgG/IgM if severe
Acute pharyngitis with oral ulceration	Herpes simplex	Swab in viral transport medium; acyclovir
	Borrelia vincentii (cause of Vincent's angina)	Swab request for Vincent's organisms; penicillin or metronidazole
Acute pharyngitis with lymphadenitis and/or skin rash	*Corynebacterium haemolyticum*	Throat swab
Unilateral tonsillar enlargement (suspected quinsy)	*Staphylococcus aureus* anaerobes & streptococci	Immediate ENT referral; co-amoxiclav *or* erythromycin & metronidazole
Pericoronitis (especially around wisdom teeth)	Streptococci & anaerobes	Amoxycillin & metronidazole or co-amoxiclav *plus* chlorhexidine mouthwash
Local trauma and possible impaction e.g., foreign body in food	Streptococci & anaerobes	Immediate ENT referral; IV amoxycillin and metronidazole
Recent travel to diphtheria-endemic areas (tropics, Russia); general toxaemia, laryngeal/pharyngeal obstruction & membrane	As above but consider *Corynebacterium diphtheriae*	Immediate hospital referral if diphtheria a possibility

Figure 6.4   Empirical therapy of acute pharyngitis

Pharyngitis & conjunctivitis	Adenovirus	Symptomatic; swab in viral transport medium
Visible oral candidosis; dentures; dry mouth syndrome; HIV risk; other immunocompromised state	*Candida albicans*	Swab and oral saline rinse for culture; miconazole gel *or* oral amphotericin B *or* fluconazole *plus* chlorhexidine mouthwash
Travel to tropical countries, systemic upset	Malaria, dengue & viral haemorrhagic fevers etc.	Immediate referral to hospital

Figure 6.4 **Empirical therapy of acute pharyngitis (continued)**

LOWER RESPIRATORY TRACT INFECTIONS

ACUTE LARYNGOTRACHEOBRONCHITIS (CROUP) & ACUTE BRONCHITIS
As these are nearly always viral, and treatment is symptomatic, attempts at virus isolation are not usually made. Severe cases may require admission to hospital when throat washings or a nasopharyngeal aspirate can be taken for viral immunofluorescence, particularly for influenza and parainfluenza viruses. If there is a rapid onset of symptoms of obstruction, epiglottitis or foreign body aspiration should be considered, especially in children, and the patient taken to hospital immediately.

ACUTE-ON-CHRONIC BRONCHITIS
Most authors do not recommend or routinely perform culture of sputum in these patients. If sputum is cultured, it consistently grows haemophili and pneumococci, and so treatment should be directed towards these organisms. Unexplained treatment failure may be related to resistant organisms and if this occurs a culture may then be appropriate so that sensitivities can be performed.

PNEUMONIA
Numerous studies have shown that the clinical distinction between classical and so-called atypical pneumonia is not as clear as previously thought.

- about 50% of cases are due to pneumococci or, less commonly, haemophili
- about 10% are caused by mycoplasmas or other 'atypical' bacteria
- 10% of infections are viral
- about 30% of pneumonias are of unknown aetiology even in studies where a wide range of investigations has been performed.

Practitioners will of course be guided in therapy by knowledge of any underlying disease and current data on epidemics of infection, but in general the guidelines on tests shown in Figure 6.6 should be useful.

SPUTUM CULTURE

These can be of value provided that the sample is not salivary and is properly coughed up. Samples should not be refrigerated but sent to the laboratory as soon as possible. As noted above, sputum culture is of little value in patients with underlying chronic bronchitis. A 'cough plate' or 'cough swab' is sometimes of use in children with cystic fibrosis if sputum cannot be obtained easily; this should be discussed with the laboratory.

BLOOD CULTURES

These are now being made available to GPs in some areas; the local laboratory should be contacted about this. If blood culture sets are available, the following are examples of indications for culture:

- high fevers (>/=39°C), or rigors

- pneumonia especially post-influenzal

- immunocompromised patient or in-dwelling Hickman line (e.g., in patients with haematological malignancy)

- diabetic patients with e.g., urinary tract symptoms, cellulitis, infected foot ulcer

- undiagnosed fever after return from tropics (NB malaria must be excluded first as a matter of urgency).

Figure 6.5   Indications for culture

The skin should first be cleaned for 30 seconds with isopropyl alcohol and allowed to dry. The needle is changed before the bottles are inoculated, and between 3 and 10 mL of blood is injected into each bottle depending on the system used; this information should be printed on the bottles.

SEROLOGICAL TESTS

In general, these require paired sera (10 mL clotted blood) 7 to 10 days apart in order to detect a rising titre of antibody although a single high titre of antibody can suggest infection with a particular agent. The laboratory will provide an interpretation of what constitutes a 'high' titre for specific organisms. Some laboratories only investigate paired sera after the second sample arrives. It is worth noting that virology laboratories store sera for several years and so a specimen taken late in the course of the illness could sometimes be matched with an old sample taken for any other reason (e.g., rubella screening in pregnancy), provided that the approximate date of the sample is known. A test for the detection of cold agglutinins is of some value for mycoplasma pneumonia although specific serology (mycoplasma IgM) should also be performed.

PNEUMONIA IN THE IMMUNOCOMPROMISED HOST INCLUDING AIDS PATIENTS

This is a complex area requiring specialist expertise and hospital referral. The management of infection caused by organisms such as pneumocystis, cytomegalovirus and aspergillus frequently involves invasive techniques for diagnostic samples, and parenteral therapy may be needed.

INVESTIGATIONS FOR COMMUNITY-ACQUIRED PNEUMONIA

Post-influenzal, post-operative or elderly patient

- blood culture if possible

- sputum culture (unless underlying chronic obstructive pulmonary disease is present)

- serology for influenza A & B in winter

Heavy smoker, middle aged to elderly (especially male), or recent travel/animal exposure

As above plus:

- serology for *Legionella pneumophila, Mycoplasma pneumoniae, Chlamydia psittaci, Coxiella burnetii* (Q fever)

- histoplasma, coccidioidomyces serology (USA / exotic travel)

- urea & electrolytes, liver function tests

Young to middle-age:

- serology for influenza, *Mycoplasma pneumoniae*, adenovirus, chlamydia (for *Chlamydia pneumoniae*)

- cold agglutinins for mycoplasma infection are sometimes useful but specific antibody studies are preferred

Child:

- normally managed in hospital but probably Respiratory Syncytial Virus (RSV), parainfluenza

Infant:

- consider *Chlamydia trachomatis*: nasopharyngeal aspirate for chlamydia.

Figure 6.6   **Investigations for community-acquired pneumonia**

Cystic fibrosis and bronchiectasis

- regular monitoring of sputum is of value to detect colonisation of CF patients with staphylococci, pseudomonas and resistant organisms including *Pseudomonas (Burkholderia) cepacia*

- some units perform aspergillus antibody screening (Radioallergosorbent test (RAST))

Immunocompromised patient including AIDS

- need hospital referral for possible bronchoscopy or empirical therapy for opportunist infection*

Pulmonary tuberculosis

- Three sputum samples taken on consecutive days

- If negative on the Ziehl-Neelsen stain, and TB is still suspected, further samples may be indicated such as a gastric aspirate or early morning urine (EMU).

*Mycobacterial blood cultures in AIDS patients for *Mycobacterium avium* complex and *Mycobacterium tuberculosis* (contact laboratory for special bottles); polymerase chain reaction (PCR) not yet available for routine diagnostic use (still under evaluation).

Figure 6.6   Investigations for community-acquired pneumonia (continued)

INTERPRETATION OF CULTURES & SEROLOGY

If pneumococci or haemophili are cultured from sputum this does not always indicate that these organisms are causing infection, but they are usually relevant if they are present in a purulent sample.

- *Moraxella catarrhalis* (formerly *Branhamella* spp.) is an opportunist commensal and is more likely to be a cause of infection in immunocompromised patients or those with underlying chest disease. Some laboratories may make a comment about the likely significance of the culture.

- *Staphylococcus aureus* and coliform bacteria are unusual sputum isolates but these organisms cause severe and fulminating disease; however, it should be noted that some patients are throat carriers of *Staph. aureus*, and antibiotic treatment predisposes to harmless colonisation with coliform bacteria.

- The management of children and young people with cystic fibrosis requires close contact between the laboratory and clinician. Sputum culture may reveal acquisition of *Staph. aureus, Pseudomonas aeruginosa* or *Pseudomonas (Burkholderia) cepacia* (particularly resistant and mucoid strains); increased sputum purulence and clinical deterioration guides the clinician's therapy since colonisation is inevitable. Also, delicate organisms such as *Haemophilus influenzae* may not be detectable on culture yet they can cause intercurrent infection.

Serological tests are specific for the detection of current infection and the clinician will be guided by the laboratory as to the significance of the results. Many people have low levels of antibody to a wide range of respiratory viruses and bacteria, and a few may react in tests for *Legionella* spp (either because they have had past infection or have cross-reacting antibodies). In the complement fixation test, antibodies against the group antigen of chlamydia are detected and so a rising titre of antibody may be due to infection with *Chlamydia psittaci, C. pneumoniae* or *C. trachomatis*. Special techniques such as micro-immunofluoresence will be needed to distinguish between the species and this is normally only done by a reference laboratory. In many serological tests, a four-fold rising titre in serum samples taken 7 to 10 days apart confirms a significant rise. For example, a rise in antibody titre from 1 in 8 to 1 in 32, or 1 in 16 to 1 in 64, is taken as significant. The reason for this stipulation is that a doubling of the titre could be due to laboratory variation in the performance of the test.

GASTROINTESTINAL TRACT INFECTIONS

OESOPHAGITIS
Pain on swallowing is rarely infective but must be considered in persons with AIDS or on immunosuppressive drugs, especially when oral candidiasis is present. Even if the mouth does not have classic features of candidiasis an oral swab plus an oral rinse (10 ml of saline) may reveal heavy colonisation.

GASTRITIS
Investigation for *Helicobacter pylori* infection should commence with a clotted blood sample for the helicobacter antibody test (usually an ELISA). The microbiology laboratory will forward it to the appropriate reference laboratory if necessary. Further tests such as the ^{14}C-urea breath test or endoscopy, biopsy and culture will, of course, have to be arranged with the local hospital.

MALABSORPTION
The main infective cause of malabsorption-type diarrhoea, especially after recent travel abroad, is giardiasis. Cysts of *Giardia lamblia*, which are passed intermittently, are seen in faeces and samples should be taken from two or three stools. Other parasites that can cause malabsorption and diarrhoea will also be detected in stools but you should request 'ova, cysts and parasites' on the form.

OTHER DIARRHOEAL DISEASE AND INFECTION
The main indications for taking faecal samples are shown in Figure 6.7:

- significant diarrhoea of any cause
- the patient is a food handler or health care worker
- the patient has returned from abroad in the past month
- the patient is immunocompromised or at high risk e.g., has sickle cell disease
- significant systemic symptoms are present
- an outbreak of diarrhoea is occurring or there is a strong association with a particular food.

Figure 6.7   Indications for taking faecal samples

All laboratories should examine faeces for salmonella, shigella, campylobacter and enterohaemorrhagic *Escherichia coli* and for other pathogens if indicated (e.g., tropical pathogens in travellers, hence the need to provide adequate information on their travel and food consumption history). Pathogens are detected in approximately a fifth of faecal samples from patients with diarrhoea but for diagnostic and public health reasons it is important that an effort is made to identify the pathogen. Ideally, three samples should be sent, taken on consecutive days, using the specially-designed faecal sample pot rather than anything else (samples occasionally arrive in the laboratory in empty crisp packets and other inappropriate containers!). About 10-20 g of sample is sufficient. In general, rectal swabs are not recommended but may be acceptable if a stool sample is unobtainable. Once the diarrhoea has resolved the sample is unlikely to yield a pathogen although in some cases it can be important to identify carriers e.g., salmonella in food handlers or sickle cell disease patients. Children with post-infectious lactose intolerance may have continued diarrhoea but infection should still be excluded, particularly to put the parents' minds at rest.

Viral infections such as those caused by rotavirus or small round structured viruses (SRSV) are detected by electron microscopy or latex agglutination. Faecal samples sent for bacteriology or parasitology can also be sent for virology if indicated on the form. Virological investigation is most appropriate for investigating outbreaks of diarrhoea in a residence or local community, rather than for sporadic episodes of infection, unless there is a strong association with shellfish consumption. Enteroviruses such as coxsackie or ECHO viruses do not cause diarrhoea but can be isolated from stools in cases of respiratory and central nervous system infection.

FOOD POISONING
The remains of food consumed at home may be submitted to the local laboratory if a patient has retained the product which was thought to have caused the problem. However, in cases related to restaurant meals or retail outlets, the local Environmental

Health Officer should be contacted through the local authority offices. It should be remembered that food responsible for cases of food poisoning often looks and tastes normal, whereas food that has 'gone off' is usually affected by environmental bacteria that do not normally cause food poisoning. Vomitus from a patient with staphylococcal food poisoning (or other toxin-mediated food-borne illness) is sometimes of investigational value, particularly when the original uneaten food sample is not available, or in cases of viral enteritis. Serological tests are rarely useful for the diagnosis of gastrointestinal infection.

PARASITE INFESTATIONS

Parasite infestations are normally readily identified by examination of a stool sample for ova, cysts and parasites, although for threadworm a portion of clear adhesive tape such as Sellotape should be applied to the anal margin then fixed to a glass slide so the laboratory can examine it for ova of *Enterobius*.

The most common worms which may be detected are shown in Figure 6.8.

If a patient is found to be infected, the rest of the family should be screened, especially for threadworm. Other worms such as hookworm and *Strongyloides stercoralis* are diagnosed by stool microscopy and may be detected in patients who have lived in endemic areas (mainly the tropics and sub-tropics). Detection of any of these worms should lead to

Infestation	Worm	Diagnosis
Threadworm/pinworm	*Enterobius vermicularis* 0.5-1.0 cm long	"Sellotape" slide applied to anal margin (3 daily samples), with microscopy for ova; faecal sample may also be useful
Roundworm	*Ascaris lumbricoides* 20-30 cm long, white smooth	Worm passed in stool or vomited; ova seen on microscopy of stool
Tapeworm	*Taenia solium* (pork) *Taenia saginata* (beef) up to 10 m long *Hymenolepis nana* (dwarf tapeworm)	Active segments 1-2 cm passed in stool ova seen on microscopy
Whipworm	*Trichuris trichuria*, 3-4 cm	Ova seen in stool

Figure 6.8   Worm infestations

treatment, usually with mebendazole (or niclosamide for tapeworms and thiabendazole for strongyloides) even if the patient is asymptomatic. Children under two years are not usually given mebendazole.

URINARY TRACT INFECTIONS

Indications for taking a urine sample for microscopy and culture are shown in Figure 6.9:

- cystitis and urethral syndrome
- pyelonephritis
- prostatitis
- suspected urinary infection in children
- assessment of patients who are permanently catheterised or practise self-catheterisation
- pregnancy (on booking/first presentation) whether symptoms are present or not
- other conditions e.g., TB, schistosomiasis
- diagnosis of infection in diabetics and immunocompromised patients even if they do not have specific symptoms.

Figure 6.9   Indications for taking a urine sample

TYPES OF SAMPLE

- mid-stream urine
- dip slide
- catheter specimen
- 'clean catch' sample (in children) (preferable to bag urine).

Notes:

- the urethral meatus should be carefully cleaned with soap and water before a sample is taken
- in catherised patients, samples should be aspirated from the tubing, not taken from the collection bag
- all samples should be tested for glucose and protein on site
- specimens should be refrigerated if they will not arrive in the laboratory within four hours, to avoid false positive results from multiplication of any contaminating urethral organisms.

Special Circumstances

- *Suspected chronic prostatitis.* Samples should be collected before and after prostatic massage.

- *Tuberculosis.* Early morning urines (the total volume) are required for suspected renal TB and when a patient suspected of having pulmonary TB cannot produce sputum or the sputum is negative for acid-fast bacilli.

Appearance of urine and spot tests

Infection is likely if any two of the following are present:

- cloudy appearance

- nitrite positive

- leucocyte esterase positive

- >5 pus cells per high powered field on microscopy

- organisms seen in non-centrifuged urine on microscopy.

Infection is unlikely if:

- urine is crystal clear **and**

- nitrite and leucocyte esterase negative, **or**

- no pus cells or organisms are seen on microscopy.

INTERPRETATION OF RESULTS

- the presence of pus cells is a reasonable guide to the presence of infection but their absence does not preclude it

- if infection is suspected in children or immunocompromised patients, full investigation is mandatory even if infection is judged unlikely on the above criteria.

CULTURE:

The original studies showed that 10^5 or more bacteria per mL of urine was clinically significant but it should be noted that this work was done on patients with pyelonephritis. Repeated isolation of a pure growth of an organism in lower numbers, e.g., 10^4 to 10^5 per mL can still indicate true infection especially in children and young women, and these days most laboratories will report smaller numbers. The 'heavy mixed growth' report means that two or more types of organism have been cultured; as true mixed infections are extremely rare, it is likely that either the culture was contaminated when taken, or there was a delay in culture which led to overgrowth of some organisms. If one of the organisms appears to predominate in the mixed culture, this is usually reported and sensitivities done. However in other cases the laboratory cannot say whether the culture is significant or not and it is inappropriate (or unsafe) to report the identity of all the organisms, and their sensitivities.

Elderly patients frequently have bacteriuria and in most cases treatment is not needed if they are well. Long-term catheterised patients always have bacteriuria, especially with unusual organisms such as *Pseudomonas* spp., and bacteriuria should not in most cases be treated unless the patient is symptomatic.

Antibiotic sensitivities

These should be provided with the report. Laboratories should be able to provide data on local antibiotic sensitivity which may help guide empirical treatment. Typical resistance rates for *E. coli* in the UK are shown in Figure 6.10.

• Ampicillin/Amoxycillin	50%
• Co-amoxiclav	15-20%
• Trimethoprim	10-15%
• Oral cephalosporin	10%
• Nitrofurantoin	10%
• Quinolones	0-2%

Figure 6.10   Typical resistance rates for E. coli in the UK

These figures do not necessarily correlate with clinical response rates in empirical therapy, and the more expensive drugs such as the quinolones and some oral cephalosporins should be reserved for difficult cases, for example when infection is resistant to treatment.

GENITAL TRACT INFECTION & HIV TESTS

Most patients who need to be investigated for sexually transmitted diseases (STDs) will attend a genito-urinary medicine clinic (or family planning clinic) where optimum techniques for diagnosis and management of STDs are available. For example, genital tract swabs, and in some cases rectal and throat swabs, are inoculated directly onto appropriate media, and rapid presumptive diagnosis of infection can be made. However, all genital tract samples sent to a microbiology laboratory from any GP, clinic or hospital department are investigated for STD pathogens, and occasionally gonococci are detected unexpectedly, e.g., in a high vaginal swabs (HVS) sent from a woman with vaginal discharge.

Swabs

- Genital tract swabs must always be placed in a charcoal transport medium.

- If gonorrhoea is suspected, cervical and urethral swabs must also be sent as the HVS is not an optimal sample for diagnosis of this infection.

- For the investigation of suspected chlamydial infection, cervical and urethral swabs are taken firmly to collect infected epithelial cells and either inoculated onto a chlamydial slide or placed in a transport medium for antigen detection (usually with an ELISA or immunofluorescence) or culture.

It is important to provide adequate information on the form. Samples from patients with a diagnosis of vaginal discharge are treated differently from those with suspected pelvic inflammatory disease or post-abortion/post-partum infection. Additional plates are inoculated for specimens from patients with these more serious diagnoses, and the interpretation of results is different (see below).

Serological Specimens

- Serological tests for genital tract infection are limited to treponemal serology for syphilis and chlamydia group antibodies; the latter is used infrequently for diagnosis.

- Gonococcal serology is no longer used.

- An ELISA test for treponemal antibody is increasingly used either as a screening test (and positive sera are then tested for VDRL/RPR & TPHA), or as a confirmatory test in place of the FTA-Abs.

- Syphilis serology can be difficult to interpret and expert advice should be sought. This is particularly important for biological false positive VDRL/RPR sera, or positive TPHA tests in persons who may have been exposed to yaws or pinta (i.e. from the Caribbean or South America respectively).

- Patients suspected of having infections such as genital herpes, lymphogranuloma venereum and chancroid should be referred to a genito-urinary medicine clinic.

TESTING FOR HIV INFECTION

HIV counsellors are available at all genito-urinary medicine clinics to advise people on the benefits or otherwise of having a test for HIV antibodies. This counselling is essential to reduce psychological morbidity after the result is available, should it be positive. (It should be unnecessary to say that testing without informed consent must never be contemplated other than in very rare and specific circumstances such as when a patient is unconscious.) If the patient is very unwilling to see a counsellor, and is perhaps a 'worried well' person who has no significant risk factors, then the pre-test counselling points shown in Figure 6.11 can be useful as a guide. In large practices and health centres it is useful if one or two individuals undergo training in HIV counselling, and AIDS awareness training for all health care professionals is available in many areas (contact the local CCDC or the genito-urinary medicine clinic).

If an HIV test is positive in the laboratory then it is repeated (with the same sample of serum) by a different method; very occasionally, a serum may need further tests at a reference laboratory. In any event, a single positive HIV test should be repeated with a fresh sample from the patient. Also, as noted in Figure 6.11, a person may have been infected only recently and will need another test after 3 to 6 months. Someone who is at continuing risk of infection ought to receive advice about safe practices in order to reduce their risk of infection, and they may need repeat tests later on.

The individual should be advised on the points given in Figure 6.11.

- confidential counselling is available in all GUM clinics

- the nature of AIDS and what the test means, with advice on risk reduction

- a negative HIV test does not mean the person will never acquire infection, and they may have recently acquired the virus but not yet become positive in the test

- insurance and finance companies may require a declaration that a test has been performed whatever the result, and this may be prejudicial to acceptance of prospective clients (from 1995 this should no longer apply)

- the implications for partners, children, or a prospective pregnancy, and confidentiality problems that may arise

- the limitations of the test and that it is not a test for AIDS but is a test for infection with the virus

- the support available, from both within and outside the health authority, for those with a positive result

- the advantages of having the test, which may help the patient with personal decisions and about changing behaviour and may help with diagnosis and treatment

- a reminder that the decision as to whether or not to have the test is solely the patient's

- the result will not be disclosed to anyone without the patient's consent. Any exceptions to this, such as when a patient is referred for treatment, should be explained.

- written information is available for consideration, and a decision about having the test can be delayed.

Figure 6.11   Points for counselling before an HIV antibody test

If the patient is a child, or is unconscious, then others may have to make the consent decision. In the event of a single exposure to HIV (e.g., rape incident; needlestick injury), further testing should be offered at 3 and 6 months.

HEPATITIS AND LYMPHADENOPATHY

- Patients with jaundice should have blood sent for hepatitis A IgM, hepatitis B surface antigen (HBsAg) and hepatitis C antibody.

- Rarer causes include cytomegalovirus and Epstein-Barr virus (an antibody test should be requested rather than a Monospot test).

- Screening of pregnant women at risk of hepatitis B is of value, particularly those from the Far East, Africa and South America since the baby is at risk of perinatally-acquired infection but can be immunised immediately after birth with immunoglobulin and vaccine. This is usually organised by the ante-natal clinic.

Prospective medical and dental students now require evidence of immunity to hepatitis B before acceptance at UK universities. They should be vaccinated (a course of three injections) without prior testing and have a clotted blood sample taken two months after the end of the course. Any non-responder (i.e. someone who has very poor or undetectable antibody) should receive a fourth vaccine dose and be re-tested a month later; if they still have not responded, they may need to be referred to an appropriate physician for further tests (e.g., anti-core IgG to detect past infection, or HBsAg) and for counselling.

Patients with an infectious mononucleosis-like illness need a Paul-Bunnell test or a Monospot test (or an equivalent latex agglutination test), with a repeated sample taken a week or two later if the first result is negative. However, if the patient has complications such as hepatitis, arthritis or a prolonged or particularly severe illness, then a clotted blood sample for anti-EBV antibody (IgG and IgM) should be sent to the virology laboratory (the Monospot test is often done in Haematology). Screening tests for cytomegalovirus and toxoplasma antibodies could also be requested on the same form if the serology does not show current EBV infection. In some cases, when high-risk behaviour for HIV is reported, a careful assessment for HIV infection is required, with pre-test counselling given by a trained counsellor .

MISCELLANEOUS SITES OF INFECTION

EYE SWABS
Patients with symptoms and signs such as photophobia, pain, corneal clouding, evidence of corneal ulceration and impaired vision, or who have had recent eye surgery or probable foreign body implantation, should be referred immediately to the nearest department of ophthalmology.

In uncomplicated conjunctivitis, indications for eye swabs are shown in Figure 6.12.

- neonatal sticky eye (consider infection with genital pathogens such as *Neisseria gonorrhoea, Chlamydial trachomatis,* as well as *Staph. aureus*)
- child or adult with persistent conjunctivitis
- contact lens wearer with acute infection
- severe recurrent blepharitis
- peri-orbital cellulitis (and refer to hospital).

Figure 6.12   Indications for eye swabs

- In general, mild conjunctivitis (especially when associated with acute coryza or another viral infections) is self-limiting and swabs are not required.

- The eye swab for bacterial culture (one from each eye) is taken from the conjunctival sac and must be placed in charcoal transport medium and transported to the laboratory within 4 to 6 hours as some organisms, such as gonococci from a neonate, can die rapidly.

- For the diagnosis of chlamydial conjunctivitis in a neonate (occasionally it occurs in adults) a scraping of the underside of the eyelid is taken after anaesthetising the eye, the material is applied to a chlamydia slide, air-dried and sent to the laboratory. Some laboratories will also require a sample of the discharge from the eye sent in their chlamydia transport medium for culture or an ELISA, but many do immunofluoresence only, on eye swabs.

- Infection with herpes simplex virus may be investigated with a swab in viral transport medium but as the symptoms and signs of keratitis are usually present (see above), the patient is normally referred to an ophthalmologist.

- Gonococcal eye infection, severe conjunctivitis that may become keratitis, anterior chamber infection and endophthalmitis, all require systemic antibiotics under expert guidance.

Eyelid lesions such as styes or mild blepharitis are not normally cultured as the results are unlikely to influence management. Eye swabs commonly grow coagulase-negative staphylococci and viridans streptococci as normal flora. Culture of coliforms and even *Staph. aureus* is common in the elderly and is not necessarily significant. If *Moraxella* spp, *Haemophilus* and pneumococci are isolated they should be treated, e.g., with topical chloramphenicol, gentamicin or fusidic acid according to the clinical setting and culture results.

EAR SWABS

- Ear swabs can be useful for the investigation of middle ear infection if pus is discharging from the ear.

- Otitis externa is usually due to *Pseudomonas* spp, although occasionally a swab yields *Aspergillus* spp, especially if the patient has received topical antibiotics. Aural toilet is more important than antimicrobials when these organisms are grown.

- Malignant otitis externa may have to be considered if *Pseudomonas aeruginosa* is cultured from an external ear swab from a diabetic patient.

- If an 'ear swab' is actually from the pinna (for example an infected ear stud) this should be stated on the request form.

SUPERFICIAL SKIN SWABS

These are only of value for the investigation of infected wounds and abscesses, or infected eczema. Boils and carbuncles are nearly always staphylococcal and do not need sampling unless they are particularly severe or if a resistant strain is likely. Patients with recurrent staphylococcal skin sepsis are often nasal carriers and a firm swab, taken high in the anterior nares, should be taken before any eradication of carriage (e.g., with mupirocin) is attempted. Always state the site of the wound as this influences the laboratory investigations and interpretation of the results. Swabs of leg ulcers are really only useful if cellulitis is present or if anaerobic infection supervenes (e.g., an offensive discharge).

Fungal infections:

- *Candida* spp can be grown from swabs or nail clippings as appropriate. Skin scrapings are made with the back of a sterile scalpel, and skin scales are collected into black paper which is then placed in a universal container. Commercial kits are also available.

Viral skin lesions such as those caused by herpes simplex virus or varicella zoster virus do not normally need to be confirmed by the laboratory but when this is required (e.g., in an immunocompromised patient) the vesicle should be lanced with a sterile needle, taking care not to cause bleeding. The fluid is placed in a small area of a glass slide and the reverse of the slide marked with a circle to indicate where the material is, and the slide is left to dry and sent off to the laboratory in a robust container similar to those used for cytology. A swab of the lanced vesicle is also taken and is placed in viral transport medium.

BIOPSIES

Biopsies for microbiological investigation need only be placed in a universal container. However if they are very small a few drops of sterile saline should be added to prevent drying during transit. Never use formalin if culture is required; if histopathological examination is also needed the biopsy must be divided or performed twice. Skin scrapings for leprosy need to be done by an experienced clinician.

MALARIA AND OTHER PARASITES

Blood should be sent in an EDTA tube to the microbiology or haematology laboratory, depending upon which one performs the test in your area. Antibody tests for malaria are not very useful, although serological tests for other parasites such as schistosoma and other worms may give strongly positive results in acute infection. Investigation for diseases such as filariasis and leishmaniasis usually require referral to a hospital for tropical diseases.

TRAVEL & OTHER SCREENING TESTS

People going abroad for their holiday or for other reasons should be advised to check at least two months in advance that they comply with the requirements of the country to be visited, and are up to date with their immunisations. The Department of Health booklet 'Health Advice for Travellers" can be obtained by patients free from travel agents, travel clinics or local authorities. A useful publication for doctors is 'Immunisation against Infectious Disease" (HMSO), published by the Health Departments. The Monthly Index of Medical Specialities (MIMS) also has travel information under the Immunisation section. Up-to-date travel advice about recent outbreaks of infectious diseases around the world can be obtained from the Communicable Disease Surveillance Centre at Colindale but only medical practitioners may use this source. Members of the public should be advised to contact a travel centre.

HEPATITIS A ANTIBODIES

The inactivated vaccine has effectively replaced passive immunisation with normal human immunoglobulin as a means of preventing hepatitis A in travellers. Normal immunoglobulin is still available commercially but it only gives protection for two months. Patients who have lived abroad as a child or who may have had hepatitis A do not need vaccine; they could be screened for antibody but this should be discussed with the local laboratory first.

HEPATITIS B ANTIBODIES

Hepatitis B vaccination for health workers and others at risk of infection comprises three doses of vaccine (0, 1 & 6 months is the standard course; 0, 1, 2 months is an 'accelerated course' in which case another dose is given at 12 months). The course must be followed by a test for serum antibody to hepatitis B surface antigen (anti-HBs) levels two months after the end of the course. Booster doses may be required some years later, depending on the result of this antibody test. The post-vaccination test for anti-HBs test is interpreted as follows:

Figure 6.13 indicates the tests for anti-HBs.

- Greater than 100 mIU/mL of anti-HBs: a good responder; five-yearly vaccination is recommended for those at continuing risk of infection.

- 10 to 100 mIU/mL of anti-HBs: a poor responder; try giving another one or two doses of vaccine to improve response.

- Less than 10 mIU/mL of anti-HBs: a poor responder and susceptible to the virus. A second course of vaccine could be tried, and new types of vaccine are becoming available to which some non-responders respond. If a healthcare worker, the individual should be advised about their work by an occupational health department. If they perform 'exposure-prone procedures' on patients then they will also need follow-up, including screening for evidence of current hepatitis B virus carriage, since such people often respond poorly to the vaccine.

Figure 6.13   Post-vaccination test for anti-HBs

Laboratories vary in their reporting of antibody levels and the above information is an example. Contact the Virologist for further guidance. In general, once an individual's response to the vaccine is established, repeated testing for anti-HBs is not required. Members of the public who have a needlestick injury in the community and who attend their GP or a casualty department are sometimes given a standard course of hepatitis B vaccine on the advice of the medical microbiologist. Antibody measurements are not required in such cases.

HIV TEST
No country should be asking for this test as a condition of entry. However, if the embassy or other official body insists, full counselling must be offered (see above).

MRSA SCREENING OF TRAVELLERS, HEALTHCARE STAFF AND PATIENTS

Figure 6.14 indicates individuals who may require screening for methicillin-resistant *Staph. aureus* (MRSA) in general practice.

- healthcare workers exposed to MRSA recently, especially if working for an agency or nursing home (hospital staff are normally checked by the occupational health department or infection control team)

- medical students and healthcare workers travelling to hospitals in other countries e.g., Australia, Canada

- patients in the community who had contact with a patient on a ward but were discharged before screening

- patients due for organ or bone marrow transplantation (usually they are screened by the transplant unit)

- patients in the community who have MRSA for the first time in a clinical specimen (e.g., a wound swab) and need to be screened for carriage at other body sites

- healthcare workers and staff in a nursing home if an outbreak occurs, if the home is not covered by their local hospital's occupational health or infection control services.

Figure 6.14   Individuals who may require screening for MRSA

- A nose and throat swab should be taken for routine screening of an individual who is being checked for carriage for any reason, but is not known to have had MRSA before.

- Healthcare workers should have the swabs taken as early as possible before they take up their post at the hospital as if they are MRSA positive, steps can be taken to eradicate the MRSA and re-screen them to confirm clearance of the MRSA.

This screening and eradication procedure could take some weeks. The local medical microbiologist or infection control nurse should be contacted for details of the procedure.

A full MRSA screen, which is performed if a staff member or patient is found to be MRSA positive on nose & throat screening, or if they have had MRSA grown from a clinical specimen, comprises repeat nose and throat swabs plus single swabs of the axillae, groin, perineum and any skin lesion such as eczema, an ulcer or other wound. Recently, residential and nursing homes for the elderly have become foci of MRSA colonisation or infection; advice should be sought from the relevant infection control personnel providing a service for the residence.

PREGNANCY

For deliveries managed in the community, screening for antibodies to rubella and syphilis are necessary although the value of the latter is doubted by some. In addition mothers at risk of hepatitis B should be screened (see 'Hepatitis' above; universal screening may be introduced in the UK in the near future). Mothers should be made aware of the availability of the HIV test should they require it. A urine sample for culture should be taken at each visit, particularly if the mother has a past history of urinary tract infection. Vaginal swabs are not of value unless active infection is suspected, or if the baby is likely to be at risk of group B streptococcal infection (preterm labour, premature rupture of membranes, fever, multiple births, diabetes, previous sibling with this disease or group B streptococcal bacteriuria).

NOTIFICATION OF INFECTIOUS DISEASES

It is the responsibility of every medical practitioner to notify certain infectious diseases when the diagnosis is made. Notifications must be timely and in some cases must be made urgently by telephone, so that investigations can be started immediately. The local CCDC or Environmental Health Officer will be able to provide details of the procedure. Figure 6.15 shows the list of notifiable infections in England and Wales. Laboratories do notify some infections when specific organisms are cultured but this does not replace the formal notification procedure.

NOTIFIABLE INFECTIONS IN ENGLAND AND WALES.

Diseases generally requiring telephone notification to a Consultant in Communicable Disease Control (CCDC) are shown in Figure 6.15.

- Anthrax
- Cholera
- Diphtheria
- Dysentery (amoebic or bacillary) in a food handler
- Food poisoning in a food handler
- Hepatitis, viral
- Leptospirosis
- Meningitis, acute
- Meningococcal septicaemia (without meningitis)
- Paratyphoid fever
- Plague
- Poliomyelitis, acute

Figure 6.15   Notifiable infections in England and Wales

- Rabies
- Relapsing fever
- Smallpox*
- Typhoid fever
- Typhus
- Viral haemorrhagic fevers (e.g., Lassa, Ebola, Marburg, etc)
- Yellow fever.

Diseases requiring only postal notification
- Dysentery (amoebic or bacillary) other than in a food handler
- Encephalitis, acute
- Food poisoning other than in a food handler
- Leprosy
- Malaria
- Measles
- Mumps
- Ophthalmia neonatorum
- Rubella
- Scarlet fever
- Tetanus
- Tuberculosis
- Whooping cough.

*still listed even though declared eradicated in 1978.

Figure 6.15   Notifiable infections in England and Wales (continued)

Chapter 7

Clinical Biochemistry

William Marshall

USES OF BIOCHEMICAL TESTS

The general principles of the use of laboratory tests in diagnosis and management have been covered in Chapter 3. However, there are some considerations that are specific to biochemical testing that it is appropriate to cover in this chapter. Later sections deal with the use (and misuse) of individual tests, and the strategies for the investigation of clinical situations that occur relatively frequently in general practice.

DIAGNOSIS

Biochemical disturbances occur frequently in disease. Some diseases, for example many inherited metabolic diseases, are due directly to a disturbance of biochemical mechanisms. In others, e.g., renal failure, biochemical disturbances arise as a result of a disorder affecting an organ or tissue with important biochemical functions. A third group comprises conditions in which biochemical changes reflect tissue damage or some other pathological process but are not specific to a particular disease. An example in the third category is the changes in plasma protein concentrations that characterise the acute phase response to acute inflammation.

Because most diseases in which measurable biochemical changes occur fall into the second and third categories, the results of single biochemical tests rarely provide a precise diagnosis. Perhaps the best example of all is the plasma sodium concentration. While severe hyponatraemia (e.g., plasma sodium concentration <120mmol/L) occurs infrequently and in a relatively small number of conditions and is usually of clinical significance, milder degrees of hyponatraemia occur frequently and in a wide variety of conditions and are often of little consequence in themselves.

Indeed, the plasma sodium concentration has been called the 'biochemical ESR', meaning that it is frequently, but non-specifically, abnormal in many patients with conditions as disparate as cancer, acute infection, chronic inflammatory diseases, etc.

But though biochemical tests, either singly or collectively (see below) rarely provide a complete diagnosis, they often provide sufficient information to enable treatment to be started, or indicate the nature of a patient's illness (e.g., that jaundice is due to biliary obstruction) to an extent that directs the rational use of other investigations.

SCREENING

Some theoretical aspects of the use of biochemical tests to detect sub-clinical disease have been discussed in chapter 3. Distinction must be made between specific screening, as in neonatal screening for phenylketonuria and congenital hypothyroidism, and the looser use of the term, implying the performance of a group (or 'profile') of tests in the hope of detecting an abnormality which may explain non-specific symptoms or of finding no abnormality and thus excluding significant disease.

In neonatal screening, the factors which determine whether a given result is regarded as positive or negative must be rigorously examined. When a panel of tests is performed, the scope for both false negative and false positive results is considerable. As has been emphasised, a test result within reference limits does not necessarily exclude disease, nor one (particularly only marginally) outside the limits imply the presence of a pathological process.

BIOCHEMICAL TESTS IN MONITORING AND FOLLOW UP

Different principles underlie the interpretation of test results in monitoring and follow up, as opposed to diagnosis, since a patient's test results will be compared with results obtained on a previous occasion rather than with reference values.

It is important to appreciate how closely related the test is to the condition in question, that is, whether a change in the test result can occur in the absence of a change in the patient's condition. Also important is the ability of the test to detect a change. This will depend on the 'critical difference' for the test (see chapter 3) and also on the closeness of the relationship between factors affecting the test and the disease itself.

Thus a significant increase (greater than the critical difference) in plasma creatinine concentration in a patient with renal impairment usually indicates progression of the condition; a similar increase in plasma urea concentration may do likewise, but could also be related to a change in protein turnover affecting the rate of production of urea independently of its excretion by the kidneys.

PROGNOSIS

Biochemical test are of limited value in assessing prognosis. The outcome of a condition is often related to many factors; the extent of any biochemical disturbance may be one of these but is often not. For example, the blood glucose concentration at the time of diagnosis of diabetes shows some correlation with the severity of symptoms, but bears none to the long-term prognosis, which depends largely on whether complications, e.g., vascular disease, develop.

DETECTION OF COMPLICATIONS

In drug trials, biochemical testing is widely used to detect unwanted side effects, e.g., hepatotoxicity. Even when a drug has an established role, such testing may still be required if side effects are a hazard (but an acceptable one given the value of the drug).

Therapeutic drug monitoring (TDM), that is, the measurement of plasma (usually) drug concentrations to determine optimal dosage, is an example of a test used to prevent, rather than detect complications.

INDIVIDUAL BIOCHEMICAL TESTS

Biochemical tests may be requested singly of in groups or profiles of related tests. The purist view might be that tests should be requested singly to answer specific questions, further tests being performed in a sequence informed by previous results until the question is answered satisfactorily. In the case of rare conditions or where technically demanding, expensive or invasive tests are required, this may prove the most efficient approach.

Biochemical tests, however, are for the most part not technically demanding, are relatively cheap and non-invasive, and it is often both convenient and more efficient to perform a group of related tests (e.g., a 'bone profile' comprising calcium, phosphate, alkaline phosphatase and albumin) at the outset of investigating a patient.

The remainder of this chapter provides a detailed summary of the biochemical tests that are most frequently requested by practitioners in primary care; discusses the grouping of some of these into profiles, and the choice of appropriate biochemical tests in frequently encountered clinical situations.

Reference ranges for enzymes can vary considerably between laboratories, these are indicated in the text with an asterix; always check reference ranges with your local laboratory.

ALBUMIN (SERUM)

- The major plasma protein.

- Involved, non-specifically, in the transport of numerous substances including unconjugated bilirubin, calcium, free fatty acids, drugs, etc.

- The most important determinant of plasma oncotic pressure (osmotic pressure due to protein) and hence of the distribution of fluid between the vascular and interstitial spaces.

Reference range	35-50g/L
Critical difference	5g/L
Sample	Whole blood preferred
Sources of erroneous results	Stasis during venepuncture can cause an apparent increase.

CAUSES OF ABNORMAL RESULTS

In general these are related to the volume of distribution and the relative rates of synthesis and breakdown/loss.

Low albumin	Poor nutrition
	Chronic liver disease
	Hypercatabolic states (e.g., sepsis, malignancy)
	Loss from gut (e.g., ulcerative colitis)
	Loss from the kidneys (especially in nephrotic syndrome)
	Over-hydration
High albumin	Dehydration

Clinical features of disorders

Low plasma albumin concentrations (usually <25g/L) may be causally associated with oedema; low concentrations can occur with oedema from other causes due to a dilutional effect. High concentrations are rare and usually iatrogenic.

Notes

- Approximately 50% of circulating calcium is bound to albumin. Most laboratory measurements of calcium measure total (free plus bound) calcium, yet only the free fraction is physiologically active. See Calcium (p.130) for details of how to assess the significance of hypocalcaemia when plasma albumin is also low.

- Low albumin concentrations can occur in many conditions, and more than one cause may be operative in an individual patient.

- In liver disease, a low albumin concentration suggests a chronic process; plasma albumin is normal in acute hepatitis.

ALBUMIN (URINE)

Normal urine albumin excretion is very low (less than can be detected by dipstick testing). Dipstick tests for protein in urine are most sensitive to albumin. False positive results occur with alkaline urine (e.g., due to bacterial contamination) and in the presence of certain antiseptics.

'Clinical' albuminuria (dipstick positive, >150mg/L) occurs in a wide variety of renal diseases and can also occur in patients with fever, following severe exercise and in urinary tract infection. Orthostatic proteinuria is proteinuria occurring only in the upright position; it is relatively common in young people. Protein should not be detectable in a sample collected while the individual is recumbent. It is probably a benign condition.

Dipstick positive proteinuria discovered incidentally, and not explicable on the basis of fever, etc., must be further investigated, initially by quantitation (24h excretion) and measurement of plasma urea/creatinine.

'Microalbuminuria' — the excretion of abnormal amounts of albumin but not detectable with dipsticks — provides a sensitive indication of incipient renal disease in patients with diabetes mellitus. Special laboratory testing is required for its quantitation.

ALKALINE PHOSPHATASE

- An enzyme, occurring particularly in osteoblasts (bone-forming cells) and the liver.

- Increased plasma activities occur in various bone and hepatobiliary diseases.

- Measured as part of bone and liver profiles.

Reference range*	25-120 IU/L (in adults; levels up to three times this may be normal in children)
Critical difference	22 IU/L
Sample	Whole blood preferred
Causes of erroneous results	None

CAUSES OF ABNORMAL RESULTS

Low levels are uncommon, and rarely of any consequence.

High levels are characteristic of bone disease associated with increased osteoblastic activity and hepatobiliary disease with partial or complete biliary obstruction.

High alkaline phosphatase due to bone disease

Paget's disease of bone

Renal osteodystrophy

Rickets, osteomalacia

Hyperparathyroid bone disease

Osteomyelitis

Healing fractures

Bone tumours (secondary and primary).

High alkaline phosphatase due to hepatobiliary disease

Cirrhosis

Hepatic tumours (secondary and primary) and other space-occupying lesions

Cholangitis

Extrahepatic biliary obstruction (e.g., carcinoma of pancreas).

Clinical features of disorders

The clinical features associated with high alkaline phosphatase levels are those of the causative condition, e.g., bone disease, liver disease, etc.

Notes

- Alkaline phosphatase is not significantly elevated in osteoporosis (unless fracture occurs), or in myeloma.

- Alkaline phosphatase is not elevated in the early stages of acute hepatitis, but may rise later.

- Elevated alkaline phosphatase can occur in late pregnancy, due to secretion of the enzyme by the placenta, and occasionally in cancer not associated with bony or hepatic involvement, due to secretion by the tumour.

- When the origin of an elevated alkaline phosphatase is in doubt, the laboratory should be able to measure the specific bone and hepatic forms of the enzyme (isoenzymes) separately.

* Reference ranges for enzymes can vary considerably between laboratories: check with your local laboratory.

ALANINE TRANSAMINASE (ALT)

(also known as alanine aminotransferase or glutamate-pyruvate transaminase, GPT).

- An enzyme, widely distributed in body tissues but present in particularly high amounts in the liver.

- Released into the plasma when there is tissue damage (e.g., hepatitis).

- ALT is a more specific indicator of liver damage than aspartate transaminase (AST) but in practice its measurement provides little information in addition to that provided by AST (see p.126) although some laboratories measure both in their panel of 'liver function tests'.

Reference range*	0-50 IU/L
Critical difference	13 IU/L
Sample	Whole blood preferred
Causes of erroneous results	None

CAUSES OF ABNORMAL RESULTS

Low levels are of no consequence but a decrease from previously elevated activities suggests a decrease in tissue damage.

High levels

- hepatitis

- cirrhosis

- cholestatic jaundice

- congestive cardiac failure (due to hepatic congestion).

Clinical features of disorders

There are no specific consequences of a raised plasma activity of ALT; associated clinical features are those of the underlying disease.

* References ranges for enzymes can vary between laboratories; check with your local laboratory.

AMYLASE

- An enzyme, present primarily in the pancreas and salivary glands.

- Its measurement is valuable in the management of the acute abdomen.

- Elevated levels of amylase can occur in many causes of this condition but clearly elevated levels are characteristic of acute pancreatitis.

Reference range   varies according to analytical method - consult local laboratory.

Critical difference   N/A

Sample   Whole blood preferred

Causes of erroneous results

Macroamylassaemia — a high plasma level of the enzyme due to its complexing with an immunoglobulin — is rare and benign.

CAUSES OF ABNORMAL RESULTS

Low levels of amylase are of no significance. In general practice, the finding of a high level in a patient with abdominal pain should prompt referral to hospital.

High levels can occur in non-abdominal conditions, e.g., acute renal failure, diabetic ketoacidosis, but are rarely a cause of diagnostic difficulty.

Note

- Measurement of amylase is of no value in the diagnosis of either chronic pancreatic insufficiency or pancreatic cancer. The levels in serum are usually normal or only slightly elevated.

ASPARTATE TRANSAMINASE (AST)

(also known as aspartate aminotransferase or glutamate-oxaloacetate transaminase, GOT)

- An enzyme, widely distributed in body tissues, occurring particularly in liver and skeletal and cardiac muscle. One of the standard 'liver function tests'.

Reference range*	0 - 55 IU/L
Critical difference	13 IU/L
Sample	Whole blood preferred
Causes of erroneous results	Measurements in haemolysed samples are invalid.

CAUSES OF ABNORMAL RESULTS

Low levels are of no consequence, but a decrease from previously elevated activities implies a decrease in tissue damage.

High levels

Liver disease: High levels occur with hepatocellular damage (i.e., hepatitis) and precede the development of jaundice. Lesser elevations are seen in cholestatic disease. Elevations up to 1-2 times the upper limit of the reference range are common incidental findings in general practice: causes include excessive alcohol consumption, obesity, drug toxicity and diabetes mellitus.

Myocardial infarction: Levels rise 12-18 hours after the onset of chest pain and may remain elevated for three days. Other causes of elevated levels include skeletal muscle damage/disease.

Clinical features of disorder: These are those of the underlying condition.

Note

- If an individual is found to have an elevated AST, there are no clinical features of liver disease, other liver function tests are normal (including no bilirubinuria) and drug effects, alcohol and obesity can be excluded, the test should be repeated after 2-4 weeks.

AUTOANTIBODIES

Autoantibodies are antibodies which react against the body's own tissues. They are classified as specific (e.g., anti-thyroid peroxidase) and non-specific (e.g., antinuclear factor). In hospitals without separate immunology departments, these antibodies may be measured in departments of chemical pathology, haematology or microbiology. Many specialised tests are available but few are of relevance to primary care; those that are include rheumatoid factor, antinuclear factor and thyroid autoantibodies.

Autoantibody results are usually expressed as a titre. This refers to the extent to which serum can be diluted and still give a positive reaction. The higher the titre (e.g., 1:256 is greater than 1:128), the greater the concentration of autoantibodies.

NON-SPECIFIC AUTOANTIBODIES
Rheumatoid factor (RhF) is an IgM antibody directed against IgG. It is detectable in significant titres (>1:128) in 75-80% of patients with rheumatoid disease. Patients with rheumatoid who are negative for RhF ('sero-negative') can usually be shown to have an IgG or IgA autoantibody but this is not detectable in standard tests for RhF.

The Rose-Waaler test refers to a specific technique (using sheep red cells coated with rabbit IgG) to detect RhF; this test tends to have lower sensitivity but greater specificity for rheumatoid disease than other tests e.g., ELISA (enzyme-linked immunosorbent assay).

The titre of RhF often, but not always, correlates with disease activity, for example falling on treatment with disease modifying drugs.

A positive test for RhF on its own is not diagnostic of rheumatoid disease, even in patients with arthropathy. Low titres of RhF are seen in a small proportion (<5%) of normal individuals, the frequency increasing with age. RhF is not specific to rheumatoid disease: it can also be positive in other rheumatic diseases (e.g., in 20-30% of patients with systemic lupus erythmatosus), and hyperglobulinaemia of any cause, e.g., sarcoidosis, myeloma and chronic (especially parasitic) infections.

Antinuclear factors (ANF) are autoantibodies which bind to nuclear material. The standard ANF test is positive in 90 - 100% of patients with systemic lupus erythmatosus (SLE). It is also positive in 20 - 30% of patients with rheumatoid disease. Positive titres can occur in the normal elderly and in association with treatment with some drugs, e.g., hydrallazine.

A range of more specific antinuclear antibody tests reacting with particular nuclear components, e.g., double stranded DNA, have been developed; these tend to show higher specificity for individual rheumatic and associated diseases.

SPECIFIC AUTOANTIBODIES
Anti-thyroid autoantibodies are present in high titres in patients with autoimmune thyroid disease. Anti-peroxidase antibodies (formerly anti-thyroid microsomal antibodies) are present in almost all patients with autoimmune hypothyroidism secondary to Hashimoto's disease. They are usually positive in Graves' disease, albeit at lower titre (<1:3200). Anti-thyroglobulin antibodies are also often detectable in these conditions. They may be positive, albeit at relatively low titre, in up to 15% of normal females and 5% of males, more frequently in the elderly.

Antibody tests are not tests of thyroid function. The detection of anti-thyroid antibodies is of no value in the diagnosis of hypo- or hyperthyroidism, but may indicate the cause of these conditions.

Antibodies to the TSH receptor are diagnostic of Graves' disease but measurement is not routinely available.

Other tissue-specific autoantibodies include antibodies against the adrenal cortex and intrinsic factor. Antibodies against red blood cells are detectable in autoimmune haemolytic anaemia.

BICARBONATE

(sometimes, more accurately, referred to as 'Total carbon dioxide' {TCO_2})

- Bicarbonate ions are the principal buffer for hydrogen ions (acid) in the extracellular fluid.

- Bicarbonate concentration tends to be low in acidosis and increased in alkalosis, unless due to a respiratory disorder.

Reference range   22-30mmol/L

Critical difference   4mmol/L

Sample   Whole blood preferred

Sources of erroneous results
Bicarbonate concentration falls when blood samples are exposed to air, due to loss of carbon dioxide. This effect can cause a significant apparent reduction in bicarbonate if a sample has to be transported to the laboratory from a remote site.

CAUSES OF ABNORMAL RESULTS
High bicarbonate

Metabolic alkalosis (e.g., prolonged vomiting, potassium deficiency)

Chronic obstructive airways disease (compensatory change).

Low bicarbonate

Metabolic acidosis (e.g., renal failure, diabetic ketoacidosis, severe cardiac failure).

Clinical features of abnormalities
Abnormal bicarbonate concentrations themselves cause no signs or symptoms; any that are present will be due to the underlying disease.

Note
- Although formerly included in many laboratories' 'electrolyte profile', bicarbonate measurements are now often not routinely available; the reasoning is that if assessment of acid-base status is required, a patient should be referred for formal measurement of arterial 'blood gases' (hydrogen ion concentration/pH, partial pressure of carbon dioxide {PCO_2} and oxygen {PO_2}), with derivation of bicarbonate from the Henderson-Hasselbalch formula.

BILIRUBIN

- An orange-yellow pigment, the end product of haem degradation, normally metabolised in the liver and then excreted into the bile.

- Accumulation causes jaundice which usually only becomes apparent when plasma concentration exceeds twice normal.

- Frequently elevated in hepatobiliary disease of any type when bilirubinuria is usually also present, and so is one of the standard 'liver function tests'.

- Haemolytic conditions can also cause elevated plasma concentrations ('pre-hepatic') but not accompanied by bilirubinuria.

Reference range	0-20μmol/L
Critical difference	10μmol/L
Sample	Whole blood preferred
Causes of erroneous results	None

CAUSES OF ABNORMAL RESULTS

High bilirubin

Hepatobiliary disease, particularly with cholestasis e.g.,

- cirrhosis (advanced)

- hepatitis (not initially)

- drug reactions (e.g., chlorpromazine, rifampicin and many others)

- hepatic metastases

- pancreatic carcinoma

- biliary strictures, etc.

- congestive cardiac failure (due to hepatic engorgement)

- haemolytic anaemias*

- pernicious anaemia*

- Gilbert's disease* (a common, benign disorder of bilirubin metabolism, causing mild, sporadic, elevations of bilirubin and mild jaundice).

*no bilirubinuria

Low bilirubin

None

Clinical features of elevated concentrations

Jaundice may be apparent to a trained observer with plasma concentrations >50μmol/L, and to a lay person if >100μmol/L. Features of the causative condition will usually be present.

Notes

- An elevated plasma bilirubin concentration is not always present in patients with hepatobiliary disease.

- Plasma bilirubin rarely exceeds 100μmol/L in haemolytic conditions in adults, or in Gilbert's disease.

- The urine does not normally contain bilirubin. Bilirubinuria is always pathological and should be tested for in any jaundiced patient. It may be detectable in hepatitis before jaundice develops.

CALCIUM

- A divalent ion which has a vital role in many physiological and biochemical processes as well as in the structure of bone.

- Calcium in the plasma is an important determinant of the excitability of nerve and muscle cells.

- Approximately half the calcium in blood is protein-bound (mainly to albumin); only the unbound fraction is physiologically active.

- Most laboratories measure total calcium but some apply a correction factor if the albumin is abnormal ('corrected calcium'). See note below.

Reference range	(total and 'corrected') 2.20-2.60mmol/L
Critical difference	0.19mmol/L
Sample	Whole blood preferred
Sources of erroneous results	Stasis during venepuncture (false elevation)

CAUSES OF ABNORMAL RESULTS

High calcium:

- dehydration (if albumin concentration increased)

- hyperparathyroidism (primary)

- malignancy (any tumour, with or without metastasis to bone, but particularly bronchial carcinoma and myeloma)

- thiazide diuretics (mild elevations only).

Low calcium:

- vitamin D deficiency (osteomalacia, rickets)

- chronic renal failure

Clinical features of disorders

Hypercalcaemia is often discovered incidentally. There are no specific clinical features. Any of the following may occur: abdominal pain, renal/ureteric colic (due to calculi), bone pain, thirst and polyuria.

Hypocalcaemia can cause paraesthesiae, muscle cramps and spasm, and, rarely, convulsions. Features of the causative condition may also be present.

Note
- The effect of an abnormal albumin concentration on total calcium can be allowed for by multiplying the measured calcium by a correction factor to give a corrected calcium.
- An approximate correction is: 'corrected calcium' = measured calcium + 0.02 x (40- plasma albumin in g/L).

CARBAMAZEPINE
- A widely used anticonvulsant drug.
- There is considerable variation between individuals in the dose required to achieve seizure control without toxicity (blurring of vision, dizziness, ataxia).
- Determining the optimum dose can be helped by monitoring plasma drug concentrations.

Reference range
Not applicable: the target range in patients treated with the drug is 17-42μmol/L (4-10mg/L).

Sample
Whole blood preferred, taken immediately before a dose (except when toxicity is suspected when a sample should be taken 3-4h after a dose).

Causes of erroneous results   None

Use of plasma measurements
- Plasma drug concentrations should always be considered in relation to the clinical circumstances.
- Some patients may have effective seizure control at plasma concentrations less than 19μmol/L; an increase in dosage is not required.
- Poor seizure control in the absence of symptoms of toxicity and plasma concentrations within the target range suggests that dosage may safely be increased.
- Plasma carbamazepine concentrations greater than 42μmol/L may be required to achieve seizure control in some patients and are acceptable if there are no features of toxicity.

CHLORIDE

- The principal negatively charged ion in the extracellular fluid.

- Chloride used to be measured routinely as part of an 'electrolyte' profile. Disturbances of chloride concentration do not occur in isolation and experience showed that its measurement rarely provided any additional diagnostic information to that provided by measuring plasma sodium concentration (the principal positively charged ion in the ECF).

- Measurement of chloride is sometimes of value in the investigation of infants with rare chloride-losing diarrhoea, and in the investigation of metabolic acidosis, but is not of any value in the diagnosis and management of patients in primary care.

CHOLESTEROL

- High plasma cholesterol concentrations are an important risk factor for atherosclerosis (especially affecting the coronary arteries).

- There is compelling evidence that lowering elevated cholesterol concentrations reduces the risk of coronary disease and reduces the risk of further events in individuals with existing disease. The decrease in risk is associated with decreased mortality.

Cholesterol circulates in the blood incorporated into particles (lipoproteins) with other fatty substances and apoproteins. The two principal lipoproteins which contain cholesterol are low density lipoprotein (LDL) and high density lipoprotein (HDL). The risk of coronary disease is associated with high levels of LDL; HDL concentrations are inversely correlated with risk, that is, are beneficial. LDL is normally present in higher concentrations and thus has the greater effect on total plasma cholesterol. Modest increases in total cholesterol above the ideal (e.g., up to 6.5mmol/L, see below) can occur due to an increase in the HDL fraction alone but greater increases are almost always due to an excess of LDL.

Reference range

The concept of a reference range for cholesterol is flawed, since increasing risk is associated within the range of concentrations seen in normal healthy individuals. The *acceptable* or *desirable* cholesterol concentration depends on the presence of other coronary risk factors (see below), but many physicians accept a total cholesterol concentration of up to 5.2mmol/L as being ideal. Higher concentrations may be acceptable in individuals who are otherwise at low risk; lower concentrations may be desirable in patients with existing coronary disease.

Ideal concentrations: total cholesterol   <5.2mmol/L

LDL cholesterol   <3.5mmol/L

HDL cholesterol   >1.1mmol/L

Critical difference	(total) 1.0mmol/L
Sample	Whole blood preferred

Sources of error

Ideally, patients should be fasted overnight before blood is taken for any lipid measurement. In practice, recent food intake has a negligible effect on cholesterol concentration but does affect triglycerides and the calculation of LDL cholesterol.

CAUSES OF ABNORMAL CHOLESTEROL CONCENTRATIONS

High total cholesterol

Genetic

- Familial (monogenic) hypercholesterolaemia (incidence 1/500)
- 'Common' or polygenic hypercholesterolaemia
- Familial combined hyperlipidaemia
- Remnant hyperlipidaemia (rare)
- Familial hyperalphalipoproteinaemia (affects HDL only).

Acquired

- Hypothyroidism
- Cholestatic liver disease
- Renal failure
- Nephrotic syndrome.

Low total cholesterol can occur in chronic illness of any type; neither a low total cholesterol, nor lowering cholesterol, is harmful.

Low HDL cholesterol

- Obesity
- Non-insulin dependent diabetes mellitus
- Physical inactivity
- Oestrogen deficiency* .

*HDL cholesterol tends to be lower in men than women, but falls in women after the menopause.

Clinical features of disorders

In addition to vascular disease, hypercholesterolaemia may cause xanthomata (cutaneous cholesterol deposits) of various types. Many patients with hypercholesterolaemia have no clinical abnormalities, but remember that the first indicator of coronary artery disease may be a myocardial infarction.

Notes

Cholesterol (and triglyceride) concentrations should be measured in patients of any age with coronary, cerebral or peripheral vascular disease, and in individuals under 60 years with the following:

- Xanthomata

- Family history of premature vascular disease

- Diabetes mellitus

- Hypertension

- Cigarette smokers.

Treatment decisions should not be based on single measurements or those made using near patient testing equipment.

Treatment of hyperlipidaemia is beyond the scope of this book but several important principles should be emphasised:

- all patients with hyperlipidaemia should be screened for possible contributory causes (e.g., hypothyroidism)

- the effects of diet and lifestyle changes should always be assessed before considering drug treatment

- a full lipid profile (including HDL cholesterol) should be obtained before starting drug treatment

- hyperlipidaemia should not be treated in isolation: appropriate intervention for other risk factors (e.g., hypertension, smoking) is essential

- the higher the overall risk of vascular disease, the lower is the desirable plasma cholesterol concentration.

Many physicians recommend drug treatment even in the absence of other risk factors if the total cholesterol remains above 7.8mmol/L even after dietary and lifestyle modification.

CORTISOL

- A steroid hormone, essential to life, secreted by the adrenal cortex under the control of anterior pituitary adrenocorticotrophic hormone (ACTH), involved in mediating the body's response to stress, maintenance of blood pressure, fluid excretion, etc.

- Plasma concentrations are increased by stress, and show a diurnal variation, being at a peak at approximately 9.00am and a trough at around midnight.

- Cortisol is usually measured as part of a dynamic test of adrenal cortical function, to diagnose adrenal failure (Addison's disease) or hyperfunction (Cushing's disease). Both these conditions are rare.

Isolated measurements of cortisol are not used in primary care. You should contact your local laboratory for advice/protocols for the investigation of suspected adrenal hyperfunction (Cushing's syndrome) or hypofunction (Addison's disease).

C-REACTIVE PROTEIN

- A marker of the acute phase response - the changes that occur in response to acute inflammation.

- Measurement of CRP is useful in the management of patients with inflammatory diseases, e.g., rheumatoid disease, Crohn's disease, to provide an early indication of an exacerbation (plasma concentration increases) or of response to treatment (decreases) and probably superior to the measurement of the erythrocyte sedimentation rate (ESR) for this purpose.

Reference range   <5mg/L

Critical difference   N/A

Sample   Whole blood required

Causes of erroneous results   None

CAUSES OF ABNORMAL RESULTS

Increased CRP

Acute inflammation

Decreased CRP

None, but the decrease of a previously increased concentration suggests resolution of the inflammatory response.

Clinical features of high CRP concentration

These are those of the underlying condition, but an increase or fall in CRP may precede any clinically detectable change.

CREATINE KINASE

- This enzyme is present in high concentrations in cardiac and skeletal muscle.

- Its major use is in the investigation of chest pain and the diagnosis and management of muscle disease.

- The cardiac isoenzyme (CK-MB) is present in higher concentration in cardiac than skeletal muscle.

Reference range*	0 - 150 IU/L
Critical difference	N/A
Sample	Whole blood preferred
Causes of erroneous results	Measurements in haemolysed samples are invalid.

CAUSES OF ABNORMAL RESULTS

Plasma levels of CK become elevated approximately 12 hours after myocardial infarction and remain elevated for approximately 48 hours. CK-MB rises earlier but not sufficiently so to direct the use of thrombolysis.

High levels are also seen after muscle trauma, in myositis, rhabdomyolysis, some muscular dystrophies and after severe or unaccustomed exercise. They may also occur in severe hypothyroidism but this is of no diagnostic value. Serial measurements are valuable in monitoring the response of patients with myositis to treatment.

Clinical features of disorders

These are those of the cause of the high CK. It should be remembered that myocardial infarction can present with syncope, confusion or left ventricular failure as well as with chest pain.

Notes

- A diagnosis of myocardial infarction should not be made, nor excluded, on the basis of CK measurements alone.

- Measurement of CK-MB is rarely indicated outside hospital practice.

- Racial variations occur for CK, with Afro-Caribbeans (particularly males) having up to twice the level of Caucasians and Asians having intermediate values.

*Reference ranges for enzymes can vary between laboratories; check with your local laboratory.

CREATININE

- A waste product of muscle metabolism, produced at a constant rate and excreted in the urine.

- Measurement in plasma is used as a test of renal function (and is superior to urea in this respect) but a normal concentration does not exclude renal impairment, especially if muscle bulk is low.

- The glomerular filtration rate must fall to approximately half normal before plasma creatinine becomes reliably increased.

Reference range	55-120μmol/L (lower in children)
Critical difference	17μmol/L
Sample	Whole blood preferred

Causes of erroneous results
Severely icteric plasma can interfere with creatinine measurement by some methods. Recent (<10h) intake of meat (especially stewed) can cause elevation of creatinine.

CAUSES OF ABNORMAL RESULTS
Low creatinine concentrations are uncommon and rarely of diagnostic significance. High concentrations are almost always indicative of renal failure.

Low creatinine
Childhood
Severe muscle wasting.

High creatinine
Renal failure (acute or chronic).

Clinical features of disorders
Creatinine is a relatively benign substance; the uraemic syndrome of renal failure is largely due to substances other than creatinine though creatinine is invariably elevated.

Notes
- Measurement of urine creatinine in a timed sample (24h or overnight) is required together with plasma creatinine to determine creatinine clearance, which provides an adequate estimation of the glomerular filtration rate for many purposes.

- Serial measurements of creatinine clearance are seldom required. If creatinine clearance is used in a patient with renal disease to assess the GFR, subsequent monitoring can be based on plasma creatinine concentration only.

- In progressive chronic renal failure, a plot of (1/creatinine) against time is usually linear.

DIGOXIN
- A anti-dysrhythmic drug with a positive inotropic action, used mainly in the management of atrial fibrillation with congestive cardiac failure.

- Toxicity (e.g., vomiting, visual disturbance, dysrhythmias) is common; its risk can be reduced by measurement of plasma concentrations.

Reference range
Not appropriate. The ideal therapeutic range is approximately 1.0-2.6nmol/L (0.8-2.0ng/mL). Therapeutic effect is minimal at lower concentrations. Clinical toxicity is almost invariable at concentrations >3.8nmol/L (3.0 ng/mL).

Sample   Whole blood preferred, taken at least six hours after the last dose.

Causes of erroneous results

Falsely elevated results may occur in patients with renal and hepatic disease, due to the presence in plasma of a poorly characterised endogenous substance - 'digoxin-like immunoreactive substance' (DLIS).

Use of plasma measurements

- when the drug is first used, and there is a poor response to treatment, or at other times if there is an apparent decrease in response

- to confirm a suspicion of digoxin toxicity

- when renal function is deteriorating (digoxin is mainly excreted in the urine)

- to determine whether continued treatment is required (if a patient's symptoms are controlled with plasma concentrations of digoxin of less than 1.0nmol/L, the drug can often safely be withdrawn).

Note

The therapeutic effect and toxicity of digoxin is enhanced by hypokalaemia and in hypothyroidism. Plasma potassium concentration must always be measured if toxicity is suspected.

DRUGS

Drugs can be measured in body fluids for a number of purposes, e.g.,

- investigation of poisoning

- suspected drug abuse

- therapeutic drug monitoring.

For the first two of these, special conditions may need to be observed before samples are collected and expert interpretation of the results of analysis are required. Patients with suspected poisoning will be referred to hospital, and those General Practitioners with a particular interest in drug abuse should liaise directly with their local laboratory to determine the service that they require. These two topics are not discussed further in this book.

All General Practitioners may be involved in therapeutic drug monitoring (TDM) — the measurement of plasma drug concentrations as an aid to determining appropriate dosage.

TDM is unnecessary for many drugs, for example because:

- a standard dose can be given safely with predictable effect (e.g., many antibiotics)

- dosage can be adjusted on the basis of clinical response (e.g., hypotensive agents)

- dosage can be adjusted on the basis of a change in a measurable parameter (e.g., hypoglycaemic drugs).

TDM is inappropriate for drugs:

- where there is a poor correlation between plasma concentration and effect.

TDM is of potential value where:

- the correlation between dosage and plasma concentration is good but there is wide variation between individuals as to the plasma concentration achieved on a particular dosage

- clinical efficacy is not easily determined (or toxicity may not easily be recognised).

In practice, TDM is valuable in the management of patients on some anticonvulsants, digoxin, lithium, theophylline (but usually only infants with recurrent apnoea and adults with severe asthma) and macrolide antibiotics (e.g., gentamicin). TDM for carbamazepine, phenytoin, digoxin and lithium is considered under separate headings. Routine TDM for other anticonvulsants, e.g., valproate, phenobarbitone, etc., is of doubtful value except in special circumstances.

GAMMA-GLUTAMYLTRANSFERASE (GGT)

- An enzyme, present mainly in the liver, often measured as part of a panel of 'liver function tests'.

- Increased plasma activities of GGT can occur in all types of liver disease but it is a particularly sensitive (though not specific) indicator of excessive consumption of alcohol.

Reference range	up to 55 IU/L*
Critical difference	40 IU/L
Sample	Whole blood preferred
Sources of erroneous results	None

CAUSES OF ABNORMAL RESULTS
High levels of GGT

- hepatitis (particularly alcoholic)

- cholestatic liver disease (of any cause)

- excessive alcohol ingestion (in the absence of hepatitis)

- treatment with certain anticonvulsant and other drugs (due to enzyme induction)

- fatty liver (e.g., in obesity, poorly controlled diabetes mellitus).

Clinical features of disorder
These are those of the causative condition.

*Reference ranges for enzymes can vary between laboratories; check with your local laboratory.

GLUCOSE
- An essential metabolic fuel.
- Glucose concentration in the blood is normally tightly controlled by the action of insulin and the 'counter-regulatory hormones' — glucagon, cortisol, catecholamines and growth hormone.
- Blood glucose concentration rises after meals and stabilises at lower levels on fasting.

Reference range	2.8-6.7mmol/L (venous blood, fasting)
Critical difference	1.6mmol/L

Sample
Blood must be collected into a tube containing fluoride and oxalate. Plasma glucose concentrations are slightly higher than blood glucose concentrations.

Sources of erroneous results
Glycolysis by red cells will consume glucose and may lower its concentration in vitro in the absence of fluoride to inhibit the process.

CAUSES OF ABNORMAL RESULTS
Low glucose
There are many causes of hypoglycaemia; the most frequent is treatment with insulin or oral hypoglycaemic drugs. Patients with hypoglycaemia due to other causes will usually require specialist investigation.

High glucose
Diabetes mellitus
Impaired glucose tolerance.

Clinical features of disorders

Hypoglycaemia can present with ataxia, confusion, behavioural disturbances, etc. (due to inadequate glucose supply to the brain) and tremor, palpitation, sweating, etc. (due to increased sympathetic activity). Hypoglycaemia should be considered in patients with a history of 'fits, faints and funny turns'.

Acute **hyperglycaemia** causes diuresis and thirst. Other features of diabetes may also be present.

Notes

- The reference range for glucose in blood is only well defined for the fasting state. Concentrations rise after meals but in normal individuals usually return to normal after two hours.

- Diabetes mellitus can be diagnosed if fasting venous blood glucose exceeds 6.7mmol/L on a single occasion in a patient with symptoms of diabetes, or on two occasions in a symptom-free individual. For a random (or post-prandial sample) the corresponding concentration is 10.0mmol/L. Diabetes should not be diagnosed on the basis of glycosuria alone.

- An oral glucose tolerance test is only required for the diagnosis of diabetes mellitus in equivocal cases; a venous blood glucose >10.0mmol/L 2h after a 75g oral glucose load is diagnostic; a value of <6.7mmol/L is normal; intermediate values are diagnostic of impaired glucose tolerance.

GONADOTROPHINS

- Luteinising hormone (LH) and follicle stimulating hormone (FSH) are anterior pituitary hormones which regulate male and female gonadal function.

- Measurement of gonadotrophins in plasma/serum can be of value (sometimes in conjunction with gonadal steroids) in suspected disorders of gonadal function.

Reference range

In women, these are dependent on the stage of the menstrual cycle; in the early follicular phase, and in men, the concentrations of FSH and LH are usually <10 IU/L.

Critical difference   N/A

Sample   Whole blood preferred

Sources of erroneous results

LH concentrations can appear very high in pregnancy and in tumours secreting chorionic gonadotrophin (hCG), due to cross reactivity between the two hormones.

CAUSES OF ABNORMAL RESULTS

Low gonadotrophins

Pituitary/hypothalamic disease (though poor sensitivity at low concentrations may make it difficult to distinguish between low and low-normal values).

High gonadotrophins

Primary gonadal failure (LH and FSH)
Azoospermia, ovulatory failure (FSH)
Polycystic ovary syndrome (LH>FSH).

Clinical features of disorders
Decreased gonadotrophin secretion may cause loss of libido, oligo- / amenorrhoea, infertility. Features of the polycystic ovary syndrome include these, plus hirsutism, obesity and insulin resistance.

Notes
- Elevated gonadotrophin concentrations with low concentrations of gonadal steroids suggests primary gonadal failure.

- Towards the menopause, FSH concentrations tend to rise before LH, although both show considerable variation. After the menopause, the concentrations of both LH and FSH are greatly elevated.

HbA1c
- A glycated (glycosylated) derivative of haemoglobin, formed at a rate dependent on blood glucose concentration.

- Its formation is effectively irreversible so that it persists for the life of the red blood cells in which it is contained.

- HbA1c is a valuable indicator of glycaemic control over the previous 4-8 weeks in patients with diabetes mellitus.

Reference range	Depends on method; typically 5% of total Hb
Sample	Anticoagulated whole blood (usually an EDTA sample)

Sources of erroneous results
With some methods, haemoglobin variants (e.g., HbF) interfere with the determination of HbA1c. In patients with shortened red cell life spans (e.g., haemolytic anaemia), HbA1c reflects glycaemic control over a shorter period than stated above.

CAUSES OF ABNORMAL RESULTS
Low levels of HbA1c do not occur.

High levels suggest poor glycaemic control; up to 7% is often taken as indicating acceptable control, and >8% poor control though this may be acceptable in elderly patients provided that they are symptom-free.

Clinical features of abnormal results
Though HbA1c binds oxygen less efficiently than normal this is not sufficient to cause any clinical disturbance, and any symptoms will be related to the diabetes or its complications.

Notes
- Measurement of HbA1c should not be used to diagnose diabetes.

- Some laboratories measure fructosamine as an index of glycaemic control. This is a measure of the glycation of plasma proteins but is generally considered to be inferior to HbA1c in monitoring glycaemic control.

- The levels quoted above are intended for guidance only. There is variation between methods and the interpretation of results and the advice of the local laboratory should be sought.

IMMUNOGLOBULINS

See section of Protein Electrophoresis p148.

LITHIUM

- Lithium salts are used for treatment and prophylaxis of uni- and bipolar affective disorders, i.e., depression and manic-depressive psychosis. In concentrations little above those required for maximum therapeutic benefit, lithium is toxic.
- It is one of the drugs for which monitoring of concentration is a valuable aid to treatment.
- As with all therapeutic drug monitoring, correct sample collection is essential if meaningful results are to be obtained.

Therapeutic range

prophylaxis: 0.5-0.8mmol/L: some younger patients may require up to 1.0mmol/L; older patients may be satisfactorily treated with levels of 0.3-0.4mmol/L.

treatment: up to 1.3mmol/L in acute mania.

Sample   Whole blood (NOT heparinized), taken 12h after last dose.

Frequency of testing

One week following initiation of treatment or any change in dosage, or should features of toxicity develop. It is usual, though probably not strictly necessary, to check serum concentrations six-monthly or annually thereafter. Creatinine and thyroid function tests (see below) should also be checked at these times.

Clinical features of toxicity

Thirst, polyuria and other symptoms are common in patients treated with lithium, even with concentrations within the ranges quoted. Benign enlargement of the thyroid, and sometimes hypothyroidism, may occur; thyroid function tests should be performed when treatment is started and then annually. Symptoms of toxicity include apathy, ataxia, tremor, vomiting and diarrhoea, which may progress to convulsions, coma and acute renal failure. Development of such symptoms should prompt urgent measurement of serum lithium concentration.

OESTRADIOL

- The principal female gonadal steroid.

- Measurements are of little use on their own but can be valuable together with measurements of gonadotrophins (p.141) in menstrual disorders, etc.

Reference range	Depends on the stage of the menstrual cycle
Critical difference	Varies according to absolute level
Sample	Whole blood preferred
Sources of erroneous results	Exogenous oestrogen administration

CAUSES OF ABNORMAL RESULTS

Low concentrations of oestradiol occur in ovarian failure of any cause (including after the menopause).

High concentrations are rare.

Notes

- Because oestrogen concentrations vary throughout the menstrual cycle, interpretation of results requires a knowledge of the stage of the cycle (if occurring). Samples taken in the early follicular phase may be the most informative.

- The value of oestradiol measurements in the diagnosis of the menopause and monitoring of oestrogen replacement treatment is not established; measurements of gonadotrophins are probably more useful. See also, **testosterone**, p.151.

PHOSPHATE

- An essential precursor of high energy phosphate compounds (e.g., ATP), component of nucleic acids, phospholipids and bone.

- Usually measured together with calcium and alkaline phosphatase as part of a 'bone profile'.

Reference range	0.8-1.4mmol/L (higher in infants)
Critical difference	0.3mmol/L
Sample	Whole or heparinised blood
Sources of erroneous results	Measurements are invalidated by haemolysis.

CAUSES OF ABNORMAL RESULTS

Isolated abnormalities of phosphate are uncommon.

Low phosphate

- Starvation
- Hyperparathyroidism
- Withdrawal from alcohol
- Renal tubular disease.

High phosphate

- Renal failure (acute and chronic)
- Bone tumours (especially metastatic).

Clinical features of disorders

Features of the cause of the abnormal phosphate concentration may be present, but unless very severe, hyper- and hypophosphataemia are usually clinically silent.

Hypophosphataemia (0.4mmol/L) can cause muscle weakness.

PHENYTOIN

- A widely used anticonvulsant drug, whose pharmacokinetics and other properties make monitoring of plasma concentrations a valuable aid to its safe and effective use.

Target range	40-80μmol/L (10-20mg/L)
Sample	Whole or heparinised blood; the time of sampling in relation to dosage is not critical.

Frequency of sampling

Three weeks should elapse after starting treatment or changing dosage before attempting to measure the plasma concentration. Once a patient has been stabilised, concentrations only require measuring if there is a deterioration in seizure control, if toxicity is suspected, or if other drugs (which may interfere with the metabolism of phenytoin) are prescribed or withdrawn. Pregnancy is a special case where regular monitoring is required.

Clinical features of toxicity

These can include nausea, vomiting, neurological disorders (e.g., nystagmus, dysarthria, ataxia) and even an increase in fit frequency.

Notes

- Symptoms of toxicity become more frequent at plasma concentrations above 80μmol/L (20mg/L) but some patients require higher concentrations to achieve seizure control and do not suffer toxicity.

- Although a lower target concentration of 40μmol/L (10mg/L) is often quoted, an increase in dose is not indicated on the basis of a low concentration alone, especially if a patient is fit-free.

For some general principles of therapeutic drug monitoring, see *Drugs*, p.138.

POTASSIUM

- Potassium is the major intracellular cation but its plasma concentration has a major effect on the excitability of nerve and muscle membranes, this being decreased in hypokalaemia and increased in hyperkalaemia.

- Frequently measured as part of a 'renal profile' e.g., 'urea (or creatinine) and electrolytes'.

Reference range	3.6-5.0mmol/L
Critical difference	0.6mmol/L
Sample	Whole blood preferred but sample *must* be freshly drawn to produce reliable results.

Sources of erroneous results

Potassium is present in high concentration in the formed elements of blood and delay in separation of cells from serum prior to analysis can lead to leakage of potassium out of cells and spurious hyperkalaemia. This can occur in the absence of visible haemolysis and is a frequent cause of apparently high potassium concentrations in patients in the primary care setting, and can cause low potassium levels to appear normal.

CAUSES OF ABNORMAL CONCENTRATIONS

Hypokalaemia (low potassium) in primary care patients is most frequently due to:

- gastrointestinal loss (diarrhoea, purgative abuse)

- renal loss (typically due to thiazide and loop diuretics).

Hyperkalaemia (high potassium), if not spurious, is most frequently due to:

- renal failure

- administration of potassium supplements/potassium-sparing diuretics, particularly in the elderly (due to decreased renal function).

Clinical features of disorders

Hypokalaemia (usually <2.5mmol/L) causes muscle weakness, decreased intestinal motility, which can lead to constipation and intestinal pseudo-obstruction, and cardiac dysrhythmias. *Hypokalaemia enhances the efficacy and toxicity of digoxin.*

Hyperkalaemia is often clinically silent but at concentrations >6.5mmol/L there is an increasing risk of cardiac arrest.

Notes

- Hypokalaemia is a frequently encountered disorder in General Practice.

- Mild hypokalaemia (<3.0mmol/L) is not usually significant (except in patients on digoxin). Renal function should be assessed before starting a patient on potassium replacement or a potassium-sparing diuretic.

- Hyperkalaemia is frequently encountered but is often artefactual (see above). If an unexpectedly elevated potassium is found (e.g., patient with normal renal function, not on potassium supplements or potassium-sparing diuretic) the level should be checked on a fresh specimen, from which the serum is separated within an hour.

PROLACTIN

- A hormone secreted by the anterior pituitary which stimulates lactation and inhibits the actions of gonadotrophins.

Reference range	50-400mIU/L
Critical difference	N/A
Sample	Whole blood required.

Sources of erroneous results
Stress increases plasma prolactin concentrations and should be avoided prior to and during venepuncture.

CAUSES OF ABNORMAL RESULTS
Low prolactin concentrations may occur in pituitary failure.

High concentrations can occur due to:

- drug treatment, especially phenothiazines, methyldopa, oestrogens
- pituitary disorders e.g., prolactin secreting tumours and other pituitary tumours
- pregnancy, lactation
- polycystic ovary syndrome
- hypothyroidism
- chronic renal failure.

Clinical features of disorders
Hypoprolactinaemia may be a feature of hypopituitarism but is rarely the sole feature. Hyperprolactinaemia is more common; it may cause loss of libido, infertility, menstrual disturbances and gynaecomastia. Prolactin-secreting tumours can present with visual disturbance, headache, etc.

Note

- Prolactin should be measured as part of the investigation of the conditions indicated above. Concentrations >5000IU/L are usually due to a prolactin secreting tumour but lower concentrations can occur with 'microadenomas' and with any of the conditions mentioned.

PROSTATE SPECIFIC ANTIGEN

- A glycoprotein secreted by the prostate which has replaced acid phosphatase as the preferred tumour marker for prostatic cancer.

- It is secreted by the normal prostate, and plasma concentrations increase with increasing age and are increased in benign prostatic hypertrophy (BPH) so that on its own it cannot be used to diagnose cancer or absence of cancer.

Reference range	<4mg/L
Critical difference	N/A
Sample	Whole blood preferred
Sources of erroneous results	None known

CAUSES OF ABNORMAL RESULTS

High PSA concentrations are characteristic of prostatic cancer. However, there is an overlap between the values seen in cancer and those in BPH or even in normal men. Thus *a high PSA on its own is not diagnostic of prostatic cancer, nor does a normal concentration exclude malignancy.*

In practice, malignancy is unlikely with a concentration <4mg/L; levels of >10mg/L are suggestive of cancer, and should prompt urgent referral to a urologist for further investigation.

Clinical features of abnormality
These are those of the causative disorder.

PROTEIN ELECTROPHORESIS

- This technique provides a visual indication of the relative concentrations of proteins and is used to detect paraproteins in serum in suspected myeloma.

- Characteristic (though non-specific) appearances occur in acute inflammation, chronic infection and protein-losing states, although the test is of little value for the investigation of these situations.

- A wide range of individual proteins can be measured in most laboratories and such measurements (e.g., of albumin, C-reactive protein) are more useful.

Reference range
Not applicable; the laboratory should provide a qualitative report and indicate the significance of any deviation from normality.

Sample Whole blood *NB anticoagulated blood (e.g., heparinised) is NOT suitable.*

Causes of erroneous results
Electrophoresis of plasma (from anticoagulated blood) will show a band due to fibrinogen, which may be mistaken for a paraprotein.

CAUSES OF ABNORMAL RESULTS
See above. Paraproteins, if present, appear as a discrete band(s). They are present in approximately 70% of patients with myeloma. Benign paraproteins occur, but the diagnosis is one of exclusion. The laboratory will advise on appropriate further investigations.

Clinical features of abnormality
Paraproteins can themselves cause various problems but these are uncommon and any clinical features associated with paraproteins are usually those of myeloma, e.g., bone pain, weight loss, anaemia, recurrent infection, renal impairment, etc. In any patient in whom a diagnosis of myeloma is entertained, other tests should include examination of an early morning urine for Bence Jones protein and full blood count.

Measurement of the concentrations of individual immunoglobulin classes (IgG, IgA, etc.) are of value in patients with myeloma, since the paraprotein can be used as a tumour marker to follow the progress of the condition. In most myelomas, the paraprotein is an IgG or IgA.

Immunoglobulin measurements may also be performed to detect deficiencies, either primary or acquired, but such patients will usually require specialist investigation.

Notes
- Either Bence Jones protein or a serum paraprotein is present in 99% of patients with myeloma.

- The finding of a high total serum protein concentration should always prompt a request for serum protein electrophoresis unless the cause is obvious. Many laboratories will perform this test automatically in such circumstances.

- Confirmation of the diagnosis of myeloma requires bone marrow examination and patients should be referred to a haematologist.

PROTEIN (TOTAL PLASMA/SERUM)
- There are over a hundred individual plasma proteins; many are present in very small concentrations.

- Approximately half the total is albumin; much of the rest is immunoglobulins (principally IgG).

- (Total protein — albumin) thus gives an approximate indication of total immunoglobulin concentration.

Reference range   60-80g/L

Critical difference   6g/L

Sample

Whole blood preferred (total plasma protein is slightly higher than total serum protein because coagulation factors are present).

Sources of erroneous results

Stasis during venepuncture can cause an apparent increase.

CAUSES OF ABNORMAL RESULTS

Low total protein concentrations can occur in:

- causes of low albumin (see p.121)

- immunodeficiency syndromes.

High total protein concentrations can occur in:

- dehydration

- hypergammaglobulinaemia, e.g., chronic infection, multiple myeloma.

Clinical features of abnormalities

A **low** total plasma protein can cause oedema due to the decreased plasma oncotic pressure (see albumin, p.121).

A **high** total protein (mainly when due to an increase in IgM in myeloma and related conditions) can cause a hyperviscosity syndrome, with e.g., confusion and cardiac and peripheral vascular insufficiency.

PROTEIN IN URINE

See Albumin (urine), p.122.

SODIUM

- The principal extracellular cation and determinant of extracellular fluid osmolality and volume.

- Abnormalities of sodium concentration can be related to abnormal water or sodium homoeostasis (or both).

- Sodium concentration is frequently measured (as part of a 'renal profile' e.g., 'urea (or creatinine) and electrolytes' but significant abnormalities of its concentration are relatively uncommon.

Reference range	135-145mmol/L
Critical difference	6mmol/L
Sample	Whole or heparinised blood
Sources of erroneous results	None of significance

CAUSES OF ABNORMAL RESULTS

There are many causes of hyponatraemia; those encountered more frequently in Primary Care include:

- chronic diuretic treatment

- chronic dilutional hypnonatraemia (also called, 'syndrome of inappropriate antidiuresis') e.g., any chronic illness

- cancer, especially of bronchus

- diarrhoea and vomiting

- congestive cardiac failure

- chronic liver disease (especially with ascites)

- chronic renal failure.

Hypernatraemia is rare in primary care; it may be seen in dehydration.

Clinical features of disorders

Hyponatraemia is often asymptomatic when mild, but severe hyponatraemia (<125mmol/L) may cause confusion, ataxia and other neurological abnormalities. Features of the causative condition may also be present.

Patients with **hypernatraemia** are usually very thirsty.

TESTOSTERONE

- The principal male sex steroid. Present in low concentrations in normal females.

- Extensively protein-bound in plasma so that total concentrations may not accurately reflect secretion and glandular activity. Some laboratories measure the plasma binding protein (sex hormone binding globulin) and report a ratio which reflects free (physiologically active) testosterone.

Reference range	9-30pmol/L (males)
	0.5-2.5pmol/L (females)
Critical difference	N/A
Sample	Whole blood preferred
Sources of erroneous results	None

CAUSES OF ABNORMAL RESULTS

Low testosterone concentrations in males suggests testicular failure; measurement of gonadotrophins (p.141) will indicate whether this is primary or secondary to pituitary disease. The further investigation and management, if appropriate, is the province of the specialist.

High testosterone concentrations in females can occur with idiopathic hirsutism, polycystic ovary syndrome and late-onset congenital adrenal hyperplasia. Concentrations >5.0pmol/L suggest a possible adrenal or ovarian tumour and must be further investigated.

Clinical features of abnormal concentrations

Low testosterone concentrations in men cause a decrease in libido, impotence, infertility, and a decrease in male secondary sexual characteristics.

High testosterone concentrations in women are associated with menstrual disturbance, hirsutism and other virilising features, and infertility.

Note
- In general, the investigation of suspected disordered gonadal function is a matter for the specialist, but the Primary Care Physician can perform simple preliminary tests and ensure both that further investigation is appropriate and that his/her patients have as much information as possible in what is often a sensitive situation.

THERAPEUTIC DRUG MONITORING
See 'Drugs' and specific entries for carbamazepine, digoxin, lithium and phenytoin.

THYROID FUNCTION TESTS
- Thyroid disease is common and thyroid function tests are frequently requested from primary care.

- Thyroid hormones (thyroxine $\{T_4\}$ and tri-iodothyronine $\{T_3\}$) are extensively protein bound in the plasma and measurements of total hormone concentrations can give misleading information if the concentrations of binding proteins are abnormal. Measurements of the free (and physiologically active) hormones (fT_4, fT_3, but particularly the former) are now replacing total hormone measurements.

- Derived indices of thyroid function, e.g., 'free thyroxine index' are now obsolete.

- Measurement of thyroid stimulating hormone (TSH) is valuable since in primary thyroid disease (which is far commoner than thyroid disease secondary to a pituitary cause), its concentration inversely reflects thyroid activity.

- Many laboratories provide a standard panel of thyroid function tests, performing additional tests as required, but to do this efficiently, adequate clinical information is essential; a frequently used panel is TSH and fT_4, with the addition of T_3 or fT_3 when hyperthyroidism is suspected.

Reference ranges*

TSH	0.3-5.0mIU/L
thyroxine (total)	60-150nmol/L
tri-iodothyronine (total)	1.2-2.9nmol/L
thyroxine (free)	9.0-26pmol/L
tri-iodothyronine (free)	3.0-8.8pmol/L
Sample	Whole blood

Sources of erroneous results

Patients with non-thyroidal illness may have abnormal thyroid function test results ('sick euthyroidism', see below) but this is uncommon in primary care. Rarely, the presence *in vivo* of antibodies to thyroid hormones may interfere with the tests and produce anomalous results.

CAUSES OF ABNORMAL RESULTS

In overt **hypothyroidism,** the TSH is typically high (may be >100 mIU/L) and fT_4 is low. In mild or early cases, TSH may be elevated but fT_4 is normal or low-normal ('compensated' or 'borderline' hypothyroidism, see notes). During treatment, fT_4 returns to normal before TSH but long term, the adequacy of replacement is indicated by a normal TSH and a normal (possibly high-normal) fT_4. During treatment, a persistently elevated TSH indicates inadequate hormone replacement, and a low TSH, excessive replacement.

Hypothyroidism secondary to pituitary failure is uncommon and rarely the presenting feature of this condition; fT_4 is low and TSH low-normal or low.

In overt **hyperthyroidism**, TSH is low (may be undetectable) and fT_4 is high; the diagnosis should be confirmed by measurement of T_3 or fT_3, which is increased. Occasionally, TSH is very low in euthyroid individuals, and in early hyperthyroidism, T_3/fT_3 may increase before the T_4 becomes frankly elevated. During successful treatment, fT_4 and T_3/fT_3 usually fall to normal before the TSH rises to normal, but long term, all results should be within their reference ranges.

Hyperthyroidism secondary to a pituitary tumour secreting TSH is exceptionally rare; both TSH and thyroid hormone concentrations are elevated.

Sick euthyroid syndrome

In patients with non-thyroidal illness of virtually any type, thyroid function tests can sometimes be misleading. The most common pattern is a low T_3/fT_3 with normal fT_4 and TSH; occasionally fT_4 is also decreased but TSH is normal. The reasons are complex and not fully understood: the consequence is that tests of thyroid function should be requested and interpreted with care in patients with other conditions.

Clinical features of disorders

The clinical features of hyper- and hypothyroidism are well described in standard texts, and patients with typical presentations rarely cause diagnostic difficulty. Nevertheless, patients reasonably suspected of having hypothyroidism on clinical grounds are occasionally found to have hyperthyroidism, and vice versa, and symptoms may sometimes only be reported in retrospect, after the initiation of appropriate treatment.

Notes

- Hypothyroidism is more common in the elderly, and is frequently insidious in onset and yet with harmful consequences. Screening, e.g., of the over 60s, is widely practised. Asymptomatic patients found to have borderline or compensated hypothyroidism should not usually be started on thyroxine replacement but must be followed up regularly, particularly if thyroid autoantibodies are present.

- Congenital hypothyroidism is screened for at the same time as phenylketonuria, a few days after birth.

- Patients treated for hypothyroidism should be followed up life long, to assess compliance and ensure the appropriateness of replacement dosage. Patients treated for hyperthyroidism should also be followed up, to detect relapse or the eventual development of hypothyroidism.

*Reference ranges may vary between laboratories: check with your local laboratory.

TOXICOLOGY

Most laboratories should be able to offer an appropriate service for patients suspected of having taken a drug overdose (e.g., paracetamol, salicylate). Others may offer a wider repertoire and all should have access to specialised Poisons Reference Units who provide information, advice, and an extensive analytical service. Their telephone numbers are in the local telephone directory.

Laboratories also measure drugs taken therapeutically and in the context of drug abuse. For information on the former, see 'Drugs' (p.138).

TRIGLYCERIDES

- Triglycerides (also called triacylglycerols) are the principal form in which energy is stored in the body: they are the major constituent of adipose tissue.

- Triglycerides circulate in the plasma as components of various lipoproteins, particularly very low density lipoproteins (VLDL) and chylomicrons (CM).

- VLDL are made in the liver, and are always present in the plasma: CM transport dietary triglyceride from the gut and are not normally present in the plasma in the fasting state.

- Triglyceride concentrations in the plasma are increased by recent food intake and when an accurate determination is required, the patient should have fasted overnight.

- High plasma triglyceride concentrations are probably an independent (of cholesterol) risk factor for coronary heart disease, albeit a far weaker one. Very high concentrations (>12mmol/L) confer a risk of pancreatitis.

- Triglycerides are usually measured together with cholesterol in 'lipid profiles'; when drug treatment is appropriate in hypercholesterolaemia, the choice of drug may be influenced by the additional presence of hyper-triglyceridaemia.

Reference range   <1.8mmol/L (fasting)

Critical difference   0.9mmol/L

Sample
Whole blood preferred. The patient should fast overnight.

Sources of erroneous results
Triglyceride concentrations are increased by recent food intake (see above).

CAUSES OF ABNORMAL RESULTS
Hypertriglyceridaemia can be due to inherited and acquired conditions:

Inherited

- familial combined hyperlipidaemia (common)

- familial hypertriglyceridaemia (uncommon)

- familial dysbetalipoproteinaemia (remnant disease, rare)

- other inherited dyslipidaemias.

Acquired

- drugs, e.g., thiazides

- corticosteroids

- diabetes mellitus

- obesity

- excessive alcohol ingestion.

Clinical features of disorders
Hypertriglyceridaemia is often asymptomatic. It may cause the plasma to appear lipaemic; its relationship to coronary heart disease has been discussed above. Pancreatitis is an uncommon, but potentially fatal, consequence of severe hypertriglcyeridaemia.

Notes

- The most severe hypertriglyceridaemia is seen in patients abusing alcohol or with poorly controlled diabetes mellitus, often superimposed on a genetic predisposition to hyperlipidaemia.

- Severe fasting hypertriglyceridaemia (>12mmol/L) merits treatment (diet and lifestyle measures with or without drugs) to reduce the risk of pancreatitis, but the management of less severe disorders can only be determined with consideration of other cardiovascular risk factors, including cholesterol.

TUMOUR MARKERS

- Tumour markers are substances secreted into body fluids or expressed on cell surfaces which are characteristic of the presence of a tumour.

- They are of potential value in screening for cancer, for diagnosis, in prognosis, in assessing the response to treatment and in long term follow up.

- In practice, the number of tumour markers of proven value in the management of malignancy is disappointingly small; there are no effective markers for the most common tumours, e.g., carcinomas of bronchus, breast, uterus and gut.

- The most frequently used tumour markers are substances secreted by tumours, and measured either in the blood or urine.

- The marker of most value in primary care is prostate specific antigen (PSA) (see p.148). Even with this marker, the sensitivity and specificity is insufficient to make its measurement alone reliable for the diagnosis or exclusion of prostatic cancer.

URATE

- Urate is the end product of nucleic acid metabolism.

- High urate concentrations can predispose to gout, due to the deposition of monosodium urate crystals in joints.

- Hyperuricaemia does not always cause gout, but gout is usually related to hyperuricaemia.

Reference range	0.2-0.4mmol/L (tends to increase with age and be higher in women than in men).
Critical difference	0.07mmol/L
Sample	Whole blood preferred
Sources of erroneous results	None

CAUSES OF ABNORMAL RESULTS

Hypouricaemia is uncommon and is of no clinical consequence.

Treatment with xanthine oxidase inhibitors (e.g., allopurinol) lowers plasma urate concentrations.

Hyperuricaemia occurs in primary (idiopathic) gout and may be due to increased synthesis or decreased excretion of urate. The only other relatively common cause in primary care is renal failure and long term treatment with thiazide diuretics.

Note

- There are many causes of arthritis, and whereas a high plasma urate concentration supports a clinical diagnosis of gout, a normal concentration does not exclude it.

UREA

- Urea is the major end product of nitrogen (protein) metabolism and is synthesised in the liver and excreted by the kidneys.

- Measurements of plasma urea concentration have in the past been the mainstay of the assessment of renal function, but the plasma creatinine concentration is more reliable.

- Plasma urea concentration increases in renal failure but can be increased in dehydration and in individuals on a high protein intake in the absence of renal impairment.

- Often measured as part of a 'renal profile' i.e., 'urea and electrolytes' — the latter meaning sodium and potassium — but creatinine provides a better index of renal function for most purposes.

Reference range	2.5-6.7mmol/L
Critical difference	2.1mmol/L
Sample	Whole blood preferred
Sources of erroneous results	None

CAUSES OF ABNORMAL RESULTS

Low plasma urea concentrations can occur in starvation but in general are uncommon.

High plasma urea concentrations occur in:

- dehydration

- renal failure

- gastrointestinal bleeding (due to catabolism of retained blood) and with recent high protein intake.

Clinical features of disorders

See 'creatinine', p.136. Urea itself is relatively non-toxic and the clinical features of the uraemic syndrome are due mainly to other substances which accumulate in renal failure.

Notes

- Plasma creatinine measurement is to be preferred to that of urea as an index of renal function (p.136).

URINALYSIS

- Dipstick testing of urine is a valuable technique in primary care, and the results may support a clinical diagnosis or point the way to further investigation. It is important that the urine sample is freshly passed.

Bilirubin

A positive test indicates an elevation of conjugated bilirubin in the plasma, indicative of hepatobiliary disease. This may precede the development of clinical jaundice.

Blood

The presence of blood in urine (if contamination e.g., with menstrual fluid can be excluded), should always be further investigated. Causes include renal disease, tumours of the urinary tract, calculi and infection.

Glucose

Glycosuria indicates either impaired glucose tolerance or a low renal threshold for glucose. Glycosuria discovered for the first time should always be followed up, initially by measurement of blood glucose.

pH

In primary care, knowledge of the pH of even a fresh sample of urine is rarely of diagnostic value.

Ketones

In a patient with insulin-dependent diabetes, the presence of ketonuria suggests incipient ketoacidosis and indicates a need for admission to hospital.

Protein

Proteinuria can occur in renal disease, urinary tract infection, or incidentally. It should always be followed up.

Urobilinogen

The presence or absence of this bile pigment from the urine is of little diagnostic significance.

Tests of value in the diagnosis of urinary tract infection are discussed in the chapter on Medical Microbiology (p.106).

PANELS OR PROFILES OF BIOCHEMICAL TESTS

It is often more informative to measure several biochemical variables at the same time. Some of the more frequently provided/requested groupings are as follows (all measurements in plasma/serum unless indicated):

LIVER FUNCTION TESTS
Total protein
Albumin
Bilirubin
Aspartate transaminase (and/or alanine transaminase)
Alkaline phosphatase
Gamma-glutamyl transferase
(Urine bilirubin).

RENAL PROFILE
Sodium
Potassium
Creatinine
(Urea)
(Total CO_2).

BONE PROFILE
Calcium
Phosphate
Alkaline phosphatase
Albumin
Creatinine

CALCULUS FORMERS
Bone profile + urate
Urine   calcium
           phosphate
           oxalate
           urate.

INFERTILITY/SEXUAL DYSFUNCTION (MALE)
Testosterone
Sex-hormone binding globulin
Gonadotrophins
Prolactin.

INFERTILITY/SEXUAL DYSFUNCTION (FEMALE)
Testosterone
Sex-hormone binding globulin
Oestradiol
Gonadotrophins
Prolactin
Thyroid function tests.

THYROID FUNCTION
TSH
Free thyroxine
(tri-iodothyronine [T_3] as appropriate, see p.152).

THE LABORATORY INVESTIGATION OF COMMON CLINICAL SYNDROMES

This section lists some of the syndromes that present frequently in general practice, in which laboratory (and particularly clinical biochemistry) investigations are of value in diagnosis and management. Conditions in which such investigation is not helpful are not given. As has been emphasised elsewhere in this book, investigations should only be requested when there is a reasonable expectation of their providing information of help in the management of the individual patient. 'Routine' requesting of tests, e.g., 'urea and electrolytes', in the absence of a specific indication is rarely helpful and can be misleading, although there are some circumstances where conditions are sufficiently common that it is worth screening for them in asymptomatic patients (p.39).

ABDOMINAL PAIN

Patients with an acute abdomen will often require referral to hospital. Laboratory investigations in patients with chronic abdominal pain are best organised in conjunction with other investigations by a surgeon or gastroenterologist.

Measurement of serum amylase (p.125) is essential in the diagnosis of suspected acute pancreatitis but is rarely indicated in General Practice. A high amylase is not unique to this condition. Right upper quadrant pain or tenderness should prompt measurement of liver function tests (p.159).

Non gastrointestinal causes of abdominal pain should not be forgotten, e.g., renal/ureteric colic, urinary tract infection, myocardial infarction, ectopic pregnancy, hypercalcaemia (rarely) and abdominal aortic aneurysm.

ANAEMIA

See pp.67-77. In the appropriate age group, the stool should be tested for the presence of occult blood.

ANTENATAL AND POSTNATAL CARE

Maternal urine should be tested for glucose and protein at antenatal visits; in many practices and hospital clinics, patients are taught to do this themselves. Hospitals screen the fetus for neural tube defects and, in high risk pregnancies, for Down's syndrome.

All babies are screened for congenital hypothyroidism and phenylketonuria at about the end of the first week of life. Capillary blood is collected from a heel prick and spotted on to special blotting paper (Guthrie cards), dried and sent to the screening laboratory. Some laboratories also screen for other conditions e.g., sickle cell disease, neuroblastoma and galactosaemia.

Neonatal screening for cystic fibrosis is not reliable. Pre-conception testing can detect a high proportion of carriers in families in whom the condition has occurred. When a couple has already had a child with cystic fibrosis, tests on the fetus early in any subsequent pregnancy have a high probability of diagnosing the condition so that the pregnancy can be terminated.

ANXIETY

This rarely has an organic cause but hyperthyroidism may need to be eliminated, especially in women, in whom it is more common. See 'Thyroid function tests', p.152.

ARTHRITIS

An elevated serum urate concentration is characteristic of gout, but many patients with hyperuricaemia do not develop gout, and gout can occur in patients with normal urate concentrations.

The white cell count may be increased both in gout and in infective arthritis but joint aspiration and examination of the fluid for crystals/evidence of infection is usually diagnostic.

Measurements of rheumatoid factor and anti-nuclear factor (p.127) are used in the diagnosis of rheumatoid disease and systemic lupus erythematosus, respectively. The ESR is non-specific. In patients with inflammatory arthritis, particularly rheumatoid, measurements of C-reactive protein (p.135) are a helpful guide to disease activity.

Some drugs used for the treatment of arthritis merit laboratory testing for efficacy (e.g., urate in patients treated with allopurinol) or toxicity (e.g., proteinuria in patients treated with pencillamine).

Laboratory tests are of no value in the diagnosis of osteoarthritis.

BACK PAIN

Laboratory investigations are of no value in patients with acute back pain.

There are as yet no reliable or widely available laboratory tests for the diagnosis of osteoporosis.

Myeloma and other malignancies should be considered in older people. For myeloma, serum protein electrophoresis (p.148) and testing of an early morning urine for Bence Jones protein are required. The ESR is usually very high but this is not a specific finding. Patients with myeloma often have a normochromic, normocytic anaemia. Less frequently (and also in other malignancies), a leukoerythroblastic anaemia may occur.

The ESR is frequently raised in patients with any cancer but there are no specific tests to screen for malignancy. In men, carcinoma of prostate may present with back pain, and measurement of prostate specific antigen (PSA) (p.148) should be requested if there are symptoms of prostatism.

BREATHLESSNESS

Anaemia should be remembered as a possible cause but otherwise, there is rarely any requirement for laboratory tests in General Practice. Measurements of arterial blood gas tensions may be vital in the management of status asthmaticus and other respiratory emergencies but are not usually available in General Practice.

BONE PAIN

A 'bone profile' (p.159) should help in the diagnosis or rickets, osteomalacia (though not osteoporosis), and Paget's disease. Typically, in rickets and osteomalacia, calcium and phosphate are low and alkaline phosphatase is high; in Paget's disease, alkaline phosphatase can be massively increased (though this can also occur, for example, with malignancy involving the hepatobiliary system) but calcium and phosphate are usually normal. These tests are usually normal in uncomplicated osteoporosis.

Primary hyperparathyroidism is a rare cause of bone pain: there is hypercalcaemia, hypo-phosphataemia (usually) and an elevated serum parathyroid hormone concentration. If vitamin D deficiency is suspected, measurement of serum 25-hydroxycholecalciferol (the most abundant metabolite of vitamin D) should be requested.

CANCER

There are no specific tests for cancer. Many patients will have non-specific abnormalities, e.g., anaemia (usually normochromic, normocytic), a high ESR, low serum albumin concentration and elevated serum alkaline phosphatase.

Tumour markers are rarely of value in the diagnosis of cancer (too many false negatives and false positives). Suspected prostatic cancer is a possible exception: men with prostatism should have PSA (prostate specific antigen, p.148) measured. A low level does not exclude cancer but a level >10mg/L should prompt urgent referral to a urologist for biopsy.

If colorectal cancer is suspected, tests for faecal occult blood (three separate samples) should be requested.

CHEST PAIN

The most widely available test for myocardial infarction is creatine kinase (CK, p135). There is considerable interest in the development of tests which will reliably diagnose myocardial infarction (or exclude the diagnosis) early enough to be of use in determining whether a patient should receive thrombolysis. At present, no generally available test will do this. Patients should be treated on the basis of a clinical diagnosis and ECG findings.

Other 'cardiac enzymes' e.g., aspartate transaminase, hydroxybutyrate dehydrogenase, which tend to increase later and remain elevated longer after a myocardial infarction, may sometimes be of value, for example in an elderly patient with an atypical presentation, e.g., confusion. It must be emphasised, however, that an increase in the activity of 'cardiac enzymes' in the serum is neither invariable in nor exclusive to, myocardial infarction.

CONFUSION

Organic causes, which may be diagnosed by appropriate laboratory tests, include: poisoning, severe electrolyte disturbance (particularly hyponatraemia), respiratory failure, renal failure and hepatic failure. Cardiac failure is another relatively common cause. Head injury should not be forgotten. The biochemical tests that may be of help are evident from the list of causes, above.

CORONARY HEART DISEASE

The diagnosis of myocardial infarction is discussed above (p.162). For the assessment of coronary risk in asymptomatic patients, measurements of plasma cholesterol (p.132) and triglycerides (p.154), ideally in the fasting state, are essential. Tests for diabetes (p.140) should be performed and, if there is hyperlipidaemia, causes such as hypothyroidism should be eliminated by appropriate tests.

DEPRESSION

Laboratory investigations rarely reveal an organic cause but endocrine disorders e.g., hypothyroidism, should be considered if there are other features of the condition. In patients requiring lithium for prophylaxis, particularly in bipolar affective disorders, therapeutic monitoring of serum concentrations of the drug is essential (p.143).

DIABETES MELLITUS

The diagnosis of diabetes is considered in the section on 'Glucose', above. Diagnosis is still sometimes delayed because of confusion between urinary frequency and polyuria.

All patients with urinary tract symptoms should have their urine tested for glucose. If glycosuria is detected, measurements of blood glucose concentration are required to determine the cause.

In patients with established diabetes, laboratory assessment of control is based on measurements of blood glucose and glycated haemoglobin (HbA1c, see p.142). The latter provides an index of long term glycaemic control (some laboratories measure fructosamine, a measure of the glycation of plasma proteins, for this purpose). Measurement of blood glucose is to be preferred to testing for glycosuria, except in elderly patients with non-insulin dependent diabetes. Assessment of renal function, lipid status and microalbuminuria (p.122) should be performed periodically, in addition to clinical assessment, e.g., ophthalmoscopy.

The detection of ketones in the urine in an unwell patient with insulin-dependent diabetes mellitus should prompt referral to hospital.

FITS, FAINTS AND FUNNY TURNS

Laboratory investigations are seldom of value. In patients with diabetes, hypoglycaemia should always be considered. Hypoglycaemia can also occur with rare insulin-secreting pancreatic tumours (insulinomas) and in association with a number of other conditions. Phaeochromocytomas (tumours of the adrenal medulla) and other rare conditions e.g., porphyria, can present in this way but the diagnosis is rarely straightforward.

The use of therapeutic drug monitoring in patients with epilepsy treated with certain anticonvulsants is discussed in a previous section (p.138).

HYPERTENSION

The extent to which patients with hypertension should be investigated is a contentious issue. The majority of patients will have essential hypertension; hypertension secondary to renal or endocrine disease accounts for fewer than 5% of cases. Nevertheless, measurement of creatinine (both to detect a possible renal cause and renal damage secondary to hypertension) and potassium (to screen for Conn's syndrome) are probably justified in all patients. Potassium must be measured before patients are started on treatment.

IMPOTENCE AND MALE SEXUAL DYSFUNCTION

Testosterone, sex-hormone binding globulin, gonadotrophins and prolactin should be measured. Diabetes should be considered: non-insulin dependent diabetes occasionally presents with impotence due to autonomic neuropathy. Both chronic renal and hepatic disease can adversely affect male gonadal function.

INFERTILITY

Once it is established that intercourse is taking place during the fertile period, semen analysis should be performed, and both partners' gonadal function investigated. If the woman is menstruating regularly, her cycles are likely to be ovulatory, but this can be checked by measuring serum progesterone on day 21. If ovulation has occurred, the concentration will often exceed 30nmol/L. Levels below 10nmol/L suggest that ovulation has not taken place. A high concentration of LH in the early follicular phase suggests polycystic ovary syndrome. High FSH and LH suggest ovarian failure. Infertility often requires specialist investigation but many apparently infertile couples will eventually conceive without intervention.

JAUNDICE

This pigmentation of the skin, mucous membranes and sclerae, is due to the deposition of bilirubin and is a consequence of an elevated plasma bilirubin concentration. Jaundice may not be apparent even to the trained observer until the plasma bilirubin concentration reaches 50μmol/L but may be obvious to the layman at concentrations greater than 100μmol/L. The appearance of jaundice may lag behind the increase in plasma concentration, and its disappearance lag behind the decrease.

All patients with suspected jaundice should have their urine tested for bilirubin. Jaundice in adults is most frequently a sign of hepatobiliary disease but can occur as a result of 'pre-hepatic' causes, e.g., haemolysis, ineffective erythropoiesis (as in pernicious anaemia). In such cases, plasma bilirubin rarely exceeds 100μmol/L and there is no bilirubin in the urine (because the excess is in the unconjugated form, which circulates bound to albumin and so is not cleared by the kidneys). Other features of the underlying condition will be present, e.g., reticulocytosis in haemolytic conditions. If bilirubin is present in the urine, the patient has hepatic or biliary disease.

In general, hepatocellular disease (e.g., hepatitis) is associated with high levels of serum transaminases whereas cholestatic disease (either intra- or extrahepatic) is associated with high levels of serum alkaline phosphatase but in some jaundiced patients, both enzymes are increased. Cholestatis can be due to intrahepatic disease (e.g., cirrhosis) or extrahepatic obstruction (e.g., carcinoma of the head of the pancreas). Biochemical tests are of little value in distinguishing between these causes.

The history and findings on examination will often allow a confident diagnosis to be made but most patients with cholestatic disease will require referral to a specialist for further investigation.

Jaundice is common in the newborn (physiological jaundice), but usually resolves rapidly and spontaneously. Specialist referral is required in all cases of jaundice due to conjugated hyperbilirubinaemia (positive urine test for bilirubin); if jaundice is present before 24 hours after birth and persists for more than two weeks; if the jaundice is rapidly deepening, or if there are any other clinical features of hepatobiliary disease.

MENSTRUAL DISORDERS
Laboratory investigations are more likely to be helpful in oligo- or amenorrhoea than in menorrhagia. The commonest cause of secondary amenorrhoea is pregnancy, and a pregnancy test should be performed however unlikely this diagnosis appears. Gonadotrophins and prolactin should be measured. Testosterone should be measured if there is hirsutism or any virilisation. The presence of clinical features of non-gonadal endocrine conditions which can cause menstrual disorders, for example hypo- or hyperthyroidism, may prompt appropriate investigations.

OBESITY
Contrary to what lay people often believe, obesity is rarely due to endocrine disease. Weight gain is a common, though not constant, feature of hypothyroidism. Obesity occurs together with hirsutism and menstrual irregularity in polycystic ovary syndrome. Cushing's syndrome is rare although a cushingoid appearance (truncal obesity, red cheeks with telangectasia, etc.) is relatively common. The best tests to exclude this condition are the measurement of 24h urine cortisol excretion and an overnight dexamethasone suppression test. The local laboratory will advise on the exact protocols for these tests.

Obesity causes insulin resistance and patients should be tested for diabetes (p.163).

OPPORTUNISTIC SCREENING
Coronary heart disease is such a major health problem that it may be justifiable to measure the serum cholesterol concentration in all adult males and post-menopausal women, in order to identify those with hypercholesterolaemia who may benefit from dietary/lifestyle advice. This is mandatory if there is a family history of premature vascular disease and is also appropriate in patients with other risk factors for cardiovascular disease, e.g., hypertension, diabetes mellitus.

Several diseases occur more frequently in the elderly, and screening healthy over 60's for these conditions may permit their early diagnosis so that treatment can be initiated before they become serious. Appropriate tests to perform include thyroid function tests (p.152), blood glucose (p.140), creatinine (p.136), a 'bone profile' and stool occult blood, together with a full blood count.

PERIPHERAL VASCULAR DISEASE
Patients with peripheral vascular disease should be investigated for hypercholesterolaemia and diabetes mellitus.

PYREXIA OF UNKNOWN ORIGIN
If an infective cause is not found, the possibility of malignancy should be considered, particularly leukaemias, lymphomas and renal adenocarcinoma. A full blood count should be performed and the urine tested for haematuria.

STROKE
Although cholesterol-lowering reduces the risk of future stroke, many patients with stroke will die of coronary heart disease and patients who survive should therefore have their serum cholesterol measured.

TIREDNESS
This common symptom can be a feature of many conditions. When investigation is considered appropriate, tests that should be done include haemoglobin, thyroid function tests, blood glucose and creatinine.

URINARY FREQUENCY/DYSURIA AND POLYURIA
In addition to tests for infection, all patients presenting with urinary symptoms should have their urine tested for glucose; if positive, blood glucose must be measured. Less common causes of polyuria than diabetes include chronic renal failure (the major complaint may be nocturia), hypercalcaemia and hypokalaemia.

In men with prostatism, prostate specific antigen (PSA, p.148) should be measured.

Patients with urinary calculi should have a bone profile and serum urate measured, together with 24h urine excretion of calcium, phosphate, oxalate and urate.

WEIGHT LOSS
Appropriate investigations will depend on what other symptoms (if any) are present. Full blood count, thyroid function tests and blood glucose are mandatory. If there are gastrointestinal symptoms, screening tests for malabsorption include a bone profile (for evidence of vitamin D deficiency) and full blood count (for evidence of haematinic deficiency). Faecal occult blood may be positive in gastrointestinal malignancy and liver function tests abnormal (typically elevated alkaline phosphatase and low albumin) if there are hepatic metastases.

FURTHER READING

Marshall WJ. Clinical Chemistry (3rd edition). London: Mosby, 1995.

APPENDIX I

GUIDELINES FOR IMPLEMENTATION OF NEAR-PATIENT TESTING

These Guidelines have been prepared by a Working Party consisting of Scientific Members of the Association of Clinical Biochemists (ACB), along with Corporate Membership of the ACB and Representation from the Royal College of Pathologists.

Scientific Members of the ACB
Dr. Danielle Freedman (Chairman)
Dr. David Burnett
Dr. Jonathan Kay
Professor Iain Percy-Robb

Corporate Member of the ACB
Mr. Alex Grant

Representation from the Royal College of Pathologists.
Dr. Trevor Gray

These notes are intended to provide helpful advice for those who are considering setting up a facility for Near-Patient Testing (analyses to be performed outside the hospital laboratory).

They are intended to help you choose the correct system for your purpose and, importantly, explain the steps required to ensure that your results are accurate and consistently reliable.

The major points you will need to consider are presented as the questions you should ask before obtaining your instrument (be it by purchase, leasing or donation), followed by answers which will help you to arrive at the correct decision.

The guidelines have the support of the Royal College of Pathologists and the Royal College of General Practitioners.

1. ANALYSES AND EQUIPMENT

• *WHAT ARE YOU GOING TO MEASURE ?*
The first step in the process is deciding which tests (analytes) you are going to perform. You should agree who will be investigated and what the total number of tests will be. This will not usually be easily established where the introduction of Near Patient Testing is a new venture.

• *WHAT EQUIPMENT IS MOST SUITABLE FOR YOUR PURPOSE ?*
There are many sources of information which can help you to reach the correct decision. These include the manufacturers and local hospitals, and other clinical laboratories.

Additional advice may also possibly be obtained from professional organisations, such as the Royal College of General Practitioners, Local Medical Committees, FHSA's and

University Departments of General Practice. The Medical Device Directorate (MDD) of the DoH has a programme of evaluation of new equipment, and publications arising from these evaluations can be sought directly from the Medical Device Directorate, 14 Russell Square, LONDON. WC1

Each analytical system has limitations, and its suitability must be assessed for the specific use to which it will be put. This use will determine the required analytical performance, throughput and costs. Recipients of the equipment need to be aware of methodological limitations, such as precision, accuracy, operating range and interferences by other substances, such as drugs. It is likely that the equipment will be operated by staff who are not trained as analysts and particular importance should be attached to the robustness of the analytical system: i.e. not what its performance is in the best conditions of operation, but rather that which will be achieved in the conditions in which it will actually be used.

Near patient testing often takes place in an environment - such as a GP clinic - where results are also being obtained from a hospital laboratory. It is important that the results from the near patient testing sites and from hospital laboratories should be comparable. Unless this is the case, interpretation will be problematic and confusion may occur if discrepant results are obtained. This may affect not only the choice of equipment, but also decisions such as the units of measurement in which the results are expressed. Early discussion with the local clinical laboratory is the best way of avoiding such problems.

- *WHAT ARE THE LIKELY COSTS ?*

The immediate cost of Near Patient Testing is determined by two main factors; the cost of the equipment and 'consumables'. The latter depends on the system chosen and may include reagents required for tests, lancets, syringes, quality control material and enrolment in supporting Quality Assurances Schemes, etc. Other overheads such as staff costs should also be included in the equation should you wish to estimate the total cost of your new test facility.

2. MAINTAINING THE EQUIPMENT

- *HOW WILL YOU LOOK AFTER THE EQUIPMENT ?*

Once the equipment is in place it will need routine maintenance. Manufacturers' instructions should be sufficient to help you achieve satisfactory maintenance and, in the event of difficulties, their Customer Services Department should provide assistance. For each item of equipment it is necessary to record its serial number, service history and a log of problems encountered in its use.

- *WHAT WILL YOU DO WHEN THE EQUIPMENT DOES NOT WORK ?*

All equipment needs planned equipment maintenance and occasional repair. The Conditions of Warranty from the supplier should be discussed with the manufacturer, and the suitability of the Service Contract should be considered. The local hospital laboratory may be able to offer service and repair. The responsibility for these should be allocated before the problems occur. It may be necessary to have a back-up procedure which may involve moving the analyses to a different item of equipment on the same site or elsewhere, such as the local hospital laboratory. This needs to be planned and agreed.

3. HEALTH AND SAFETY

• *WILL YOU BE ABLE TO INITIATE AND MAINTAIN THE REQUIRED HEALTH & SAFETY PROCEDURES ?*
All procedures involving patients and biological tests require strict adherence to professionally acceptable health & safety standards.

The safety of the patient must always be assured. This entails hygienic methods of obtaining samples of blood and performing tests. Some patients may feel faint when blood is being taken. Therefore either a chair or a couch should be provided. Staff should be trained in the appropriate First Aid procedures.

Care must be taken to ensure that the biological hazards which can arise from tests using human blood or body fluids do not put operating staff or others at risk. This requires the formulation of Safety Procedures covering operational methods, the disposal of 'sharps' and body fluids, and the routine decontamination of equipment and working surfaces. If required, specialist microbiological advice will be available from your local hospital laboratory or the Public Health Laboratory Service on these matters. Advice on potential electrical or chemical hazards, including COSHH (Control of Substances Hazardous to Health) procedures should be followed and can be obtained from either the manufacturer or the local hospital laboratory.

It is possible that the sites intended for specimen collection and analyses may not have been specifically designed for this purpose. Particular aspects - in addition to those previously mentioned - which need to be considered are physical security, confidentiality of reports and the legal requirements of the Data Protection Act. These considerations are particularly important when the site is also going to be used for other purposes.

4. PERSONNEL REQUIREMENTS

• *WHAT PARTICULAR SKILLS WILL THEY NEED ?*
The skills which are needed by the staff include patient preparation, specimen collection, chemical analysis and recording and interpretation of results. It will be necessary to review aspects of Health & Safety and the maintenance of equipment. These tasks may be carried out by one person or distributed between several. Specimen collection will most commonly be by finger-prick or venepuncture. The member of staff who collects the specimen needs to be trained in the appropriate response to adverse reaction, such as faints, and possibly in First Aid.

• *HOW WILL THE STAFF BE TRAINED ?*
It is beyond dispute that well trained staff help to ensure high quality test results. All manufacturers should be able to assist in providing comprehensive training to cover operational, interpretative and follow-up activities which will help you achieve the desired quality. This process should cover in-service training of existing staff, the induction of new staff and routine refresher training across all involved personnel. In all cases training should be tailored to the background and experience of the person concerned. The individual responsible for the training should be clearly identified. They may be an existing member of staff, the manufacturer or an outside body such as the local hospital

laboratory. It is good practice to record all training procedures and conclusions as these could be used in determining staff responsibilities in Near-Patient Testing.

5. QUALITY ASSURANCE

• *CAN YOU TRUST YOUR REPORTS ?*

One of the most important aspects of quality assurance is that equipment is clean, well maintained and operated, and results recorded according to a standard procedure. Confidence that results from hospital based clinical laboratories are reliable comes from such procedures.

Although these are well understood and taken very seriously in laboratories, they have sometimes been omitted when analyses are introduced elsewhere.

There are two components of analytical Quality Assurance: *Internal Quality Control* and *External Quality Assessment*.

Internal Quality Control is a means of checking that results are reliable before they are issued. In order to do this, samples with known concentrations of the analyte are run through the usual procedure. The key features of a scheme are the frequency with which the checks will be performed, the material that will be used, the recording of the results and the rules which determine acceptable performance. It is good practice for the outcome to be reviewed by someone other than the analyst. Even with the best current schemes these procedures do not check all stages in the production of reports and their limitations should be understood.

External Quality Assessment differs in that its findings are not available until after the results have been issued. It allows confidence that the results are not varying over time, that they are similar to those obtained at other sites and, ideally, with other equipment and analytical approaches. It involves analysis of samples received from an external source. External Quality Assessment schemes may be operated by the manufacturer of the equipment or reagents, by external bodies such as the Wolfson Laboratories in Birmingham, or by the local hospital laboratory.

• *HOW WILL THE RESULTS BE RECORDED ?*

Quality Assurance also requires that recording of data is satisfactory.

It is necessary to record the following:

    i. Name of patient

    ii. Date and time of the analysis

    iii. Results obtained

    iv. Batch number of reagents being used

    v. Name of operator

For the individual tested this may involve the recording of age, sex, location and general practitioner. Additional information may include whether the individual was fasting and details of drug treatment.

It is necessary to record this information for use by other healthcare professionals and for the purposes of clinical review, workload analyses and audit. It may also be required for legal purposes at any time in the future. The permanent record must be able to support all of these functions.

It is possible that results of tests may be compared with those coming from elsewhere, such as local hospital laboratories. This makes it important to record the source of each result. Reports should include unit of measurement and may include a reference range. Reports may be stored on paper (which should be a bound volume, rather than loose sheets), a dedicated computer or a computer used for other functions, such as a GP system or an Occupational Health system. For each of these, you should decide how long the reports will be kept and who will have access to them. If reports are to be issued, the format should be agreed and each report should include its source.

6. INTERPRETATION OF RESULTS

• *WHO WILL BE RESPONSIBLE FOR THE INTERPRETATION OF RESULTS ?*

Near Patient Testing has two features which can increase the pressure on whoever is responsible: the results are available more quickly and the patient is still present. Once reliable results have been produced, they can then be interpreted to influence patient care. If the results are to be interpreted by someone other than the patient's medical practitioner, then guidelines for interpretation and advice should be defined in advance. These guidelines may include other factors which need to be considered, and whether other healthcare professionals are to be involved in the case of abnormal results.

• *WHO WILL SUPPLY EXPERT HELP IN INTERPRETATION ?*

You may need support in arranging further clinical advice, which may be sought from your local hospital laboratory, or in the solving of analytical problems, this may also be sought from your local hospital laboratory staff or the manufacturers of the equipment. It is likely that support will be more readily offered if the criteria for referral have been agreed in advance.

FURTHER READING

Safe working and the prevention of infection in clinical laboratories Health Services Advisory Committee. HMSO 1991.

Safe working and the prevention of infection in clinical laboratories; model rules for staff and visitors. Health Services Advisory Committee. HMSO 1991.

HN (Hazard) (87) 13. Blood glucose measurements; reliability of results produced in extra-laboratory areas.

Guidelines to Good Practice: Outstationing of Diagnostic Equipment. Appendix 6 of 'Review of pathology services staffing: A report to the manpower planning advisory group.' Management Advisory Service to the NHS.

Quality assessment of blood glucose monitors in use outside the hospital laboratory. Drucker, R.F., Williams, D.R.R., Price, C.P.J. Clin. Pathol. 1983; 36: 948-953.

Consumer Protection Act 1987. See Bulletin of the Royal College of Pathologists No. 67, June 1989, p 8-9.

Essential considerations in the provision of near-patient testing facilities. Marks, V. Ann. Clin. Biochem. 1988; 25: 220-225.

Organisation and quality control of extra-laboratory blood glucose measurements. Price, C.P., Burrin, J.M., Nattrass, M.Diab. Med. 1988; 5: 705-709.

Quality of plasma cholesterol measurements in primary care. Broughton, P.M.G., Bullock, D.G., Cramb, R. BMJ 1989. 298: p 297-298.

Desktop laboratory technology in General Practice Stott, N.C.H. BMJ 1989; 229: 579-580.

The use of diagnostic equipment outside the diagnostic laboratory (1990). Evans, S.J., McVittie, J.D., Kay, J.D.S., Oxford Regional Health Authority.

The Control of Substances Hazardous to Health Regulations 1988.

'Guidelines on the control of Near-Patient Tests (NPT) and procedures performed on patients by non-Pathology Staff' (1993). Available from D Kelshaw, Secretary, Joint Working Group on Quality Assurance c/o Mast House, Derby Road, Liverpool, L20 1EA.

HN (Hazard) (89) 31: 'Blood Gas Measurements: The need for reliability of results produced in extra-laboratory areas'

APPENDIX II

SUMMARY OF PROCEDURE FOR SENDING HIGH-RISK SPECIMENS TO PATHOLOGY DEPARTMENTS OR FOR REQUESTING VENESECTION BY A PHLEBOTOMIST

All specimens should be placed in plastic bags (e.g., 'kangaroo' bags) with the form in a separate compartment. There are certain exceptions, e.g., outlying clinical areas with special transport arrangements, formalinised histopathology samples and 24-hour collections. In the paragraphs below, **risk of infection** means a high probability of infection associated with recognised risk behaviour, unless recently negative for markers of infection.

HEPATITIS B & C, NON-A NON-B HEPATITIS RISK

Label form and specimen 'Hepatitis-risk' or 'Danger of Infection'; give antigen/antibody status if known (state if not known). Place form and specimen in separate compartments of a double-compartment polythene bag.

HIV RISK

HIV-risk patients will be bled by a phlebotomist provided warning information is given on the request form (see note on confidentiality below).

Label form and specimen 'Danger of Infection', and write 'HIV-risk' on the form; place the form and specimen in separate compartments of a double-compartment polythene bag.

CONFIDENTIALITY: If necessary, place the form in a brown envelope and label it with the laboratory destination and hazard stickers.

VIRAL HAEMORRHAGIC FEVERS INCLUDING LASSA FEVER

This includes individuals with an unexplained fever returning from Africa within the previous three weeks, especially if they have been in rural areas. Take a Sequestrene sample for malaria parasites and mark the form 'PUO, recently in Africa'; the sample should be taken to Haematology where the blood films will be prepared and disinfected. (NB suspected falciparum malaria must be dealt with urgently). Other blood specimens may be taken but should be retained in the room until the risk of Lassa Fever is discounted (unless very urgent analysis is required). Notify the Medical Microbiologist on call if transfer of the patient to an Isolation Unit is required.

OTHER e.g., TB, TYPHOID, BRUCELLA

Label form and specimens 'Danger of Infection'. Write the suspected diagnosis on the form. Place form and specimen in separate compartments of a double-compartment polythene bag. Blood samples from TB patients do not have to be specially labelled.

APPENDIX III

INFECTION CONTROL POLICY FOR GENERAL PRACTITIONER'S SURGERIES

INTRODUCTION

The following precautions have been designed to protect staff and patients from cross-infection. Particular attention is drawn to the changes in practice which have been brought about by the advent of the inoculation-risk viruses, including the human immunodeficiency virus (HIV) and hepatitis B & C. There has been a tendency to try to identify clients or patients who might have these viruses and use elaborate precautions when treating them. As it is not possible to identify all carriers it is sensible to introduce a system of universal precautions whereby high risk procedures are identified rather than high risk individuals. If staff use the recommended precautions this should protect them from inoculation risks, such as sharps injuries and splashes onto mucous membranes.

Staff have a responsibility to their patients, their colleagues and themselves to maintain good working practices. Their general personal health and hygiene is also important; for example, skin and respiratory infections can be transmitted to others.

All staff should be able to locate the equipment for dealing with spillages and first aid, and be familiar with the parts of this policy which apply to them.

1. **Blood and body fluids**
   All staff must handle safely body tissue, fluids, specimens, sharps and needles from any procedure on any patient. Safe handling of body fluids and tissues means wearing gloves if hands are likely to become contaminated with body fluids, such as dealing with used dressings or bedpans. Safe handling of used sharps and needles means immediate disposal into a sharps disposal bin (see below). To avoid unnecessary handling, storage and transporting of blood and to avoid inappropriate use of the practice nurse's time it is recommended that patients are sent for blood tests to a hospital phlebotomy department (or use a local phlebotomy service if available).

2. **Sharps containers**
   Discard sharps only into approved sharps containers. Never fill sharps containers more than three-quarters full. Never leave needles and sharps lying around for other staff to clear away. Each person is responsible for the safe disposal of sharps they have used. Needles should not be resheathed, bent or broken — but if resheathing is unavoidable (for particular types of needle/syringe units) a safe, one-handed technique should be used.

3. **Spillages of blood and body fluid**

   Spillages must be dealt with immediately. The spillage is covered with chlorine-releasing granules (e.g., Haz-Tab Granules, Guest Medical, Edenbridge, UK); alternatively, ordinary household bleach diluted 1 in 10 can be used: this represents 1% hypochlorite (1 in 10,000 ppm available chlorine), and it is poured onto paper towels laid on the spillage. Chlorine tablets made up in water according to the manufacturer's instructions can also be used (e.g., Haz-Tabs, Guest Medical). The room should be kept well ventilated, and also the area must be clearly demarcated (e.g., with hazard tape) so that others don't slip on the spillage or contaminate themselves. After 30 minutes, the spillage has been disinfected and the remaining fluid is cleared away with more paper towels by a member of staff wearing gloves and a plastic apron. Residual bleach can leave a white deposit so rinsing with water may be necessary. The gloves, plastic apron and paper towels should be discarded into a yellow bag for incineration.

   If **broken glass** is also present in the spillage, glass **must not** be picked up with hands even if the individual is wearing gloves as clinical gloves do not protect against sharp objects; a scoop made of plastic or cardboard must be used, after the disinfection period has elapsed. Sharps such as broken glass must be placed in a designated sharps bin for incineration.

   1% hypochlorite and hypochlorite granules are strong and may give off chlorine fumes if mixed with a large volume fluid spillage such as urine; in such cases, the bulk of the fluid should be mopped up first by a trained member of staff wearing protective clothing, as described above, and then the contaminated floor area or surface disinfected. Finally, diluted bleach should be made up fresh on the day of use from the concentrated product, as it deteriorates rapidly. A dilute solution of bleach (0.1%, i.e., 1 in 100 neat bleach) can be used for daily cleaning of surfaces which may have become lightly contaminated with body fluids, e.g., a section of bench used for urine testing, or for receiving and preparing laboratory samples.

It is not difficult to make up a spillage kit for the surgery, and the following components are suggested:

- a strong plastic box with a well-fitting lid
- bleach granules and / or tablets
- paper towels
- latex gloves and plastic pinafore
- a plastic scoop for broken glass
- a small plastic sharps container if not available elsewhere in the surgery or suite

- a yellow plastic bag for incineration

- yellow warning tape labelled 'Biohazard' or 'Danger of Infection' to demarcate the area

- clear instructions.

Alternatively, ready-made kits are available through commercial suppliers.

4. **Protective clothing**

   Disposable gloves and plastic aprons are required for all procedures where a healthcare worker may be exposed to body fluids, e.g., pelvic examination, urine testing and changing dressings of exudating wounds. Unless they have skin problems, in which case gloves must be worn, experienced practitioners may use their discretion about wearing gloves for venepuncture, as manual dexterity may be impaired by gloves. Sterile gloves are only required for procedures where the hands come into contact with sterile tissues as in some types of minor surgery. Broken skin on the hands must be covered by a waterproof plaster. Disposable items must be discarded into a yellow bag after use — gloves should be changed between patients, but plastic aprons may be worn for more than one procedure as long as they look perfectly clean.

   It is important to remember that cross-infection could occur when protective clothing such as gloves are worn and that body fluid contamination of notes, surfaces and other individuals could occur if gloves are not removed after the procedure is finished. White coats and other uniforms should be kept clean.

5. **Linen**

   Blankets should not be used as an underlay for couches. Curtains, overblankets and pillow cases should be changed whenever they become visibly soiled or contaminated. Pillows should have a plastic cover under the pillow case; the case should be washed whenever it becomes soiled, and changed whenever it is damaged. If the pillow itself becomes soiled it should be cleaned or replaced. Paper sheeting should be used to cover couches, including the pillow, changed between patients, and discarded into a yellow bag for incineration.

   Disposable quilted pads can be placed on the couch for comfort and where procedures are to be performed in the pelvic region, e.g., a vaginal examination.

6. **Disinfectants**

   Household detergent and hot water are adequate for all cleaning purposes, for example chairs, couches and other fittings. A chlorine disinfectant is needed for decontamination after body fluid spillages (see above). In addition, dressing trolleys and worktops for clinical procedures should be wiped over with 70% industrial methylated spirit or ethyl alcohol before and after use. Ordinary soap, in liquid or bar form, is adequate for most purposes and kinder to skin. 'Hibisol' handrub should also be available at handbasins for procedures where extra hand disinfection is required - for example before performing minor surgery or after contamination with body fluids.

A freshly-prepared solution of hypochlorite may be used in certain situations for soaking heat sensitive, re-usable items: see item 7.5.

7. **Sterilising instruments**

Used instruments should not be left on worktops, in handbasins or lying around. Where a CSSD service is available instruments should be bagged, labelled and placed in the designated container for collection. Where washing and sterilising takes place on site the following points must be observed:-

7.1 **Boilers do not sterilise**. They are effective for disinfecting articles which are not for use on sterile tissue e.g., most bowls, gallipots, speculae and forceps used in general practice.

7.2 **Steam steriliser benchtop autoclaves** must be correctly installed, regularly maintained and only used by staff who have been taught their safe operation. The manufacturer's instructions should be clearly displayed. It is recommended that a named member of staff should be responsible for all training and record-keeping in connection with these machines. A common mistake is to wrap instruments before they are placed in bench-top autoclaves (see below).

7.3 **Used instruments** A safe system must be implemented for storing used instruments awaiting cleaning and disinfection/sterilisation, such as a covered bowl of detergent or a bucket lined with a plastic bag which can hold all the instruments from a series of procedures e.g., Family Planning Clinics. Alternatively, it may be more convenient to place each instrument in a receiver and remove it to the washing area between patients. Washing should take place at a designated sink, using a chlorine-releasing disinfectant 10,000 ppm (i.e. bleach diluted 1 in 10) with added detergent. A plastic apron and heavy duty rubber gloves must be worn and care taken not to splash fluids. Gloves and cleaning brushes must be kept scrupulously clean and dry between sessions and discarded as soon as they become damaged.

7.4 **Items such as coil packs** must be processed **unwrapped** in bench top sterilisers to ensure complete penetration by the steam. If they are to be removed from the steriliser and stored before use they should be left open for sterilisation, then wrapped in foil (using a sterile technique) and put through the process again prior to storage.

7.5 **The use of glutaraldehyde solutions** is not recommended in GP surgeries; it is a health hazard unless used with proper ventilation. Items which cannot be sterilised by heat should be disposable, e.g., practice caps. If there are difficulties in obtaining enough of these items it is permissible to use a hypochlorite solution. The solution **must be changed daily** and made up according to the manufacturer's instructions. Items must be **scrupulously clean** before they are completely immersed in the solution for at least an hour. They should be rinsed and dried before use.

8. **Waste disposal**

   Household and office rubbish may be discarded in the normal way. Waste generated during clinical procedures should be placed in yellow bags for incineration. Aerosol cans and glass items must not be sent for incineration. All 'sharps' e.g., needles, blades, broken glass etc. must be disposed of into sharps containers. Yellow bags and sharps bins must be securely fastened before placing at the designated collection point in accordance with your local policy.

9. **Specimens**

   Patients should be equipped with the correct containers and specimen bags for taking their own samples. Receptionists should have a supply of specimen bags at the desk so that patients who arrive without one can drop their sample straight into the bag. If a leaky sample is put on the desk it should be treated as a spillage — see section 3 above. See section 4 for advice on venepuncture.

10. **Babies**

    Parents should change nappies and carry out any necessary toilet. A clean paper sheet should be placed on the weighing scales for each baby. Wash the scales thoroughly with soap and hot water if they become contaminated with faeces. The scales should be wiped over with hot soapy water at the start of each session.

11. **First Aid**

    In addition to the usual selection of dressings and waterproof plasters there should be an eyewash bottle (chemists stock preparations for this purpose) and a Laerdal airway to avoid the need for giving direct mouth-to-mouth resuscitation.

12. **Inoculation accidents**

    If staff members do not have access to an occupational health service, one of the practice doctors must take named responsibility for care and counselling of staff who accidentally inoculate themselves through a needlestick injury or splash of body fluid into mucous membranes. In the event of an accident:

12.1 Wash the site with soap and water or use the eyewash.

12.2 Encourage bleeding.

12.3 Note details of the client from whom the sample came and obtain a 10 ml sample of blood for urgent HBsAg status; contact the local microbiology or virology department.

12.4 Report to the appropriate GP, an occupational health department or the nearest Accident and Emergency Department.

Further advice may be obtained from:

Consultant in Communicable Disease Control at the local Department of Public Health

Consultant Microbiologist (Infection Control Doctor) at the local hospital

Control of Infection Senior Nurse at the local hospital

Out of hours: Duty Medical Microbiologist (Senior Registrar or Consultant) via the local hospital switchboard.

Main Index

Laboratory Tests Index

Disease (Disorder) Index

A

Abdominal pain, 160
Acral lentiginous melanoma, 56
Actinic keratosis, 47, *50*
Acute bronchitis, 99
Acute cervical lymphadenopathy, 95
Acute laryngotracheobronchitis, 99
Acuteonchronic bronchitis, 99
Addison's disease, 135
Adenovirus infection, 96
Adrenal disease, 135, 152
AIDS, 102
Albuminuria, 122
Alcohol, excess, 75, 139, 145
Anaemia, 69-77, 160
Anaemia of chronic disease, *71, 74-75*
Angiofibroma, 49
Antenatal testing, 116, 160
Anxiety, 161
Aortic aneurysm, 160
Arthritis, 161
Atherosclerosis, 132
Autoimmune thyroid disease, 127

B

Back pain, 161
Basal cell carcinoma, 48, *50*
Basal cell papilloma, 49
Benign acquired nevus, *52, 54*
Benign juvenile melanoma, 54
Bleeding, 87
Blue nevus, 54
    cellular, *53, 54*
Bone disease, 123, 124, 159
Bone pain, 162
Bone tumours, 145
Bowen's disease, 48, *50*
Breathlessness, 161

Bronchiectasis, 102
Bronchitis, 99
Bruising, 87

C

Cancer, 156, 162
    see also specific headings
Carcinoma-in-situ, 48, *50*
Cellular blue nevus, *53, 54*
Cervical cancer, 57-62
Cervical intraepithelial neoplasia, 58-60
Cervical lymphadenopathy, acute, 95
Chancroid, 109
Chest pain, 162
Chlamydia trachomatis, 101
Chronic myeloid leukaemia, 79
Chronic obstructive airways disease, 128
Colorectal cancer, 162
Confusion, 162
Congenital adrenal hyperplasia, 152
Coronary heart disease, 163, 165
Croup, 99
Cushing's disease, 135
Cystic fibrosis, 102, 103, 160
Cystitis, 106
Cytomegalovirus, 111

D

Dehydration, 130, 150, 157
Depression, 163
Dermatofibroma, 49, *52*
Diabetes mellitus, 106, 140, 142-143, 163
Diphtheria, 96
Dyslipidaemia
    see Cholesterol, Triglycerides
Dysplastic nevus, 55
Dysuria, 166